ON THE JOB:
The Essentials of Nursing Assisting

Second Edition

ON THE JOB:
The Essentials of Nursing Assisting

Second Edition

Barbara R. Hegner
(deceased)

Barbara Acello
Independent Nurse Consultant and Educator

Prepared by Janine Anderson, BSN, RN
Revised for the 10th ed. by Barbara Acello

DELMAR
CENGAGE Learning   Australia Brazil Canada Mexico Singapore Spain United Kingdom United States

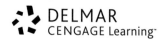

DELMAR
CENGAGE Learning

On The Job: The Essentials of
Nursing Assisting
Second Edition
Barbara R. Hegner and
Barbara Acello

Vice President, Health Care
Business Unit:
William Brottmiller

Director of Learning Solutions:
Matthew Kane

Managing Editor:
Marah Bellegarde

Acquisitions Editor:
Matthew Seeley

Product Manager:
Jadin Babin-Kavanaugh

Editorial Assistant:
Megan Tarquinio

Marketing Director:
Jennifer McAvey

Senior Marketing Manager:
Lynn Henn

Marketing Manager:
Michele McTighe

Marketing Coordinator:
Chelsea Iaquinta

Technology Director:
Laurie Davis

Technology Product Manager:
Mary Colleen Liburdi

Technology Project Manager:
Carolyn Fox

Production Director:
Carolyn Miller

Content Project Manager:
Kenneth McGrath

Senior Art Director:
Jack Pendleton

For product information and technology assistance, contact us at
Cengage Learning Customer & Sales Support, 1-800-354-9706

For permission to use material from this text or product,
submit all requests online at **cengage.com/permissions**
Further permissions questions can be emailed to

Library of Congress Control Number: 2007020187

ISBN-13: 978-1-4180-6612-3

ISBN-10: 1-4180-6612-5

Delmar Cengage Learning
5 Maxwell Drive
Clifton Park, NY 12065-2919
USA

Cengage Learning products are represented in Canada by Nelson Education, Ltd.

For your lifelong learning solutions, visit
delmar.cengage.com

Visit our corporate website at **www.cengage.com**

Notice to the Reader
Publisher does not warrant or guarantee any of the products described herein or perform any independent analysis in connection with any of the product information contained herein. Publisher does not assume, and expressly disclaims, any obligation to obtain and include information other than that provided to it by the manufacturer. The reader is expressly warned to consider and adopt all safety precautions that might be indicated by the activities described herein and to avoid all potential hazards. By following the instructions contained herein, the reader willingly assumes all risks in connection with such instructions. The publisher makes no representations or warranties of any kind, including but not limited to, the warranties of fitness for particular purpose or merchantability, nor are any such representations implied with respect to the material set forth herein, and the publisher takes no responsibility with respect to such material. The publisher shall not be liable for any special, consequential, or exemplary damages resulting, in whole or part, from the readers' use of, or reliance upon, this material.

Printed in Canada
2 3 4 5 6 7 8 12 11 10 09 08

CONTENTS

PREFACE

On the Job is a handbook for students and nursing assistants in the clinical setting. It is designed to provide rapid answers to questions likely to be asked during practice. The transition from classroom to workplace can be overwhelming as learned procedures and knowledge are applied to the care of a patient. It is often helpful to have a reference for ready access to the definitions of forgotten words, reminders of critical actions in patient care, or the signs and symptoms of a common condition. *On the Job* is the perfect reference for nursing assistants.

Having the Answers

Nursing assistants are important members of the health care team. You are privileged to be entrusted with the care of patients in private, personal, and very vulnerable situations. You make many valuable contributions to the patients' safety, security, and well-being. You are the eyes and ears of the nurses, and the services you provide are valuable to them. Nursing is both an art and a science, and nursing service workers are generalists. Nursing assistants learn a vast amount of general knowledge about many subjects, and this knowledge sustains you when you are on duty.

All of the information in this book is relevant to nursing assistants in clinical practice, but the information may not be committed to memory. For this reason, the book is a convenient size that is designed to be carried to work in a pocket or purse. The information in this revision is specialized, and likely to be needed in clinical practice. Having the ability to quickly find essential elements in a pocket guide will make you feel confident and secure, especially when you are gaining experience.

Your general knowledge will sustain you in most patient care situations, but there will be times when you need to research to find information for specialized patient care situations. This is a positive activity: Never feel ashamed for not having all the answers. None of us knows them all. Caring about your patients and taking time to look for accurate information is commendable and helps you adhere to high standards of care.

About Your Book

On the Job: Essentials of Nursing Assisting was written using current clinical information that will complement more exhaustive sources of patient care and nursing reference material. This book was developed to be a reference guide of up-to-date information that will help you survive and thrive in the ever-changing health care facility environment. It is not meant to be an exhaustive or comprehensive source of patient care information, such as a textbook.

New Information

Successful nursing assistants are well organized, with good communication skills. New information in this revision will help you to manage your time wisely, enabling you to get the job done with fewer steps and less frustration.

New content has been added to reflect the industry trends in pain recognition and management, as well as general comfort, rest, and sleep measures. Introductory information has been included for working in the home health care industry, and preparing a nursing bag, which is the toolkit used by nursing assistants who work in home care.

Obesity has become a major public health issue in the United States. It is a complex, misunderstood condition with many causes. This serious, chronic condition is a factor in five of the ten leading causes of death. Approximately one in three American adults is obese, so a chapter has been added on caring for bariatric (obese) patients. This is a new health care specialty, and many hospitals have specialized bariatric care units. Obese persons experience social discrimination and have many physical problems. An understanding of their needs and how to meet them is essential in today's health care environment. The nursing assistant and the patient are at risk of injury during routine patient care. Although your facility may not have a special bariatric unit, you will encounter obese patients in general clinical practice in hospitals and long-term care facilities. Knowing how to safely and efficiently care for and meet their highly specialized needs is a important, rewarding responsibility.

Finding the Information

On the Job: Essentials of Nursing Assisting was designed to make the material easy to find. The format consists of many short, concise narratives, charts, lists, and tables so that you can readily access and apply or implement the information. Information is grouped together in logical format that will enable you to quickly locate the information about subjects for which the nursing assistant is accountable. Section headings and content listings will assist you in finding the information quickly. Everything is important. Determining which subject is the most important would be impossible.

Suggestions and Comments

In the author's opinion, the patient is the most important individual in the facility. This book was written with the belief that *the nursing assistant is the most important worker in the facility.* Properly motivated and educated nursing assistants are important for the well-being of patients and the overall operation of the facility. You are a key member of the team and will receive a great deal of personal satisfaction from your job. Delmar Cengage Learning is committed to helping you succeed by providing quality educational materials and tools to prepare you for your job responsibilities as a member of the health care team. Feel free to contact me with your suggestions and comments through Delmar Cengage Learning or via e-mail to bacello@spamcop.net.

VITAL SIGNS

When a patient first enters a facility, a baseline set of vital signs is taken. This enables nursing staff to compare subsequent readings and to identify changes.

TEMPERATURE

Selecting the Temperature Measurement Site

Refer to Table 1-1. Once a site for measuring temperature is selected, it should be used for subsequent readings unless the patient's condition changes and a different site has to be used. Remember that there is a difference between the readings from different sites. Record the site that has been used after the reading.

Normal Temperature Variation

A patient's body temperature will normally vary by 1 to 3°F. It is lowest in the morning and higher in the afternoon and evening.

Report any deviation from normal to the nurse.

See Figure 1-1 and Tables 1-2 and 1-5.

Tympanic Temperatures

The tympanic temperature is used routinely in many facilities. It is the fastest, most convenient, and most economical method, but it can also generate inaccurate readings if the user's technique is not precise. Ear thermometers are similar to cameras: They provide the temperature of what

Table 1-1	ADVANTAGES AND DISADVANTAGES OF TEMPERATURE MEASUREMENT SITES	
ROUTE	ADVANTAGES	DISADVANTAGES
Axillary	Safe Easily accessible Noninvasive	The thermometer must be held in place for 10 minutes. Least accurate reading.
Oral	Convenient Comfortable	Takes 3 minutes to get an accurate reading. Young children or uncooperative, coughing, confused, irrational, and restless patients can break the thermometer. Someone who has a chill or has a history of epilepsy may also break the thermometer.

(continues)

Table 1-1 ADVANTAGES AND DISADVANTAGES OF TEMPERATURE MEASUREMENT SITES (CONTINUED)

ROUTE	ADVANTAGES	DISADVANTAGES
		Should not be used when the person is unconscious or very weak.
		Should not be used when the patient has had oral surgery or has a mouth infection.
		Not reliable after the patient has been eating, smoking, or drinking or is receiving oxygen (except nasal prongs).
		Should not be used if the patient is a mouth breather.
		May provide a false reading if the patient wears dentures.
Rectal	Some experts consider this the most accurate measurement.	Takes 3 minutes to get a reading; thermometer must be held in place.
		Does not respond to changes in body temperature as quickly as an oral temperature.
		Inconvenient and unpleasant for patient. Requires lubrication.
		The thermometer may be embedded in feces, causing inaccurate values. It should be placed against the wall of the rectum.
		Should not be used in newborns, patients with heart attack, in a patient following rectal surgery, in those who are uncooperative, or in those with convulsive disorders.
Tympanic	Easily accessible	Ear wax or ear infection can alter reading.
	Convenient	Patient has to remove hearing aids.
	Can provide an accurate reading of body core temperature	Have to wait 15 minutes if patient has been outside or has been lying on the ear that is to be used.
	Quick measurement (takes a few seconds)	Should not be used in patients who have had ear surgery.
	Noninvasive	Proper technique must be used to avoid inaccurate readings.

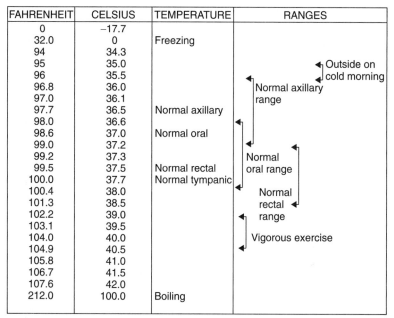

Figure 1-1 Average temperatures and ranges.

Table 1-2	AVERAGE TEMPERATURES IN INFANTS AND CHILDREN
AGE	TEMPERATURE
3 months	99.4°F
6 months	99.5°F
1 year	99.7°F
3 years	99.0°F
5 years	98.6°F
9 years	98.1°F

Table 1-3	NORMAL RANGES FOR TYMPANIC TEMPERATURES	
YEARS OF AGE	FAHRENHEIT	CELSIUS
0–2	97.5–100.4°F	36.4–38.0°C
3–10	97.0–100.0°F	36.1–37.8°C
11–65	96.6–99.7°F	35.9–37.6°C
>65	96.4–99.5°F	35.8–37.5°C

you point them at. If the thermometer is not used correctly, you get an inaccurate reading. To ensure an accurate reading, insert the probe tip into the ear as far as it will go. Next, rotate the probe until it is aligned with the jaw. Quickly press the "scan" button. If you suspect an inaccurate value, double-check your technique and take the temperature again. Several common problems can cause inaccurate readings.

- The detector at the end of the thermometer is not flat against the tympanic membrane.
- The scan button is pressed before the probe is fully inserted.
- A probe cover is used more than once.
- A thermometer is used without a probe cover.
- The lens of the thermometer is improperly cleaned.
- The manufacturer's instructions for placing the probe tip into the ear are not followed; following instructions for the thermometer you are using is important.
- A thermometer's lens is broken or missing; the lens is the shiny disc at the end of the probe tip through which the infrared energy must pass to be processed.

- The patient is in a cold area or is being fanned, or the thermometer has been stored in the flow of cold air and did not warm up before being used.
- The thermometer is set to maintenance mode. In this mode, the LCD read-out screen reads "CAL" or something similar, indicating it is being used for calibration or other bench work.
- If the patient is a child, the position of the probe tip does not point at the midpoint between the eyebrow and sideburn on the opposite side of the face.
- If the patient is an adult, the thermometer is not aligned with the jaw.
- If the patient is an adult, the pinna of the ear was not pulled up and back to straighten the ear canal.

When Your Patient is an Infant or Child

The nursing assistant must become familiar with "best practices" for monitoring vital signs on infants and children. "Best practices" for taking vital signs in infants and children are listed in Table 1-4.

Table 1-4   "BEST PRACTICES" FOR TAKING VITAL SIGNS IN INFANTS AND CHILDREN

- Check with the nurse before taking a rectal temperature on a *newborn infant*. In some facilities, the first rectal temperature must be taken by the nurse to ensure the rectum is patent. Sometimes a child is born with one end of the intestines closed. Surgical correction is required.
  - After the nurse or physician determines that the anus is patent, the rectal method may be safely used. However, in many facilities, axillary or tympanic temperatures are the method of choice for newborn infants.
  - A typical policy is to check and record the newborn infant's axillary temperature every 30 to 60 minutes until stable, then every 4 hours or according to the nurse's instructions.
  - When taking a rectal temperature, grasp the infant's ankles gently, but firmly, with one hand. Cover the penis of a male infant with a diaper. Insert

Table 1-4   "BEST PRACTICES" FOR TAKING VITAL SIGNS IN INFANTS AND CHILDREN (CONTINUED)

the lubricated thermometer into the rectum while holding the ankles. Continue to hold the ankles with one hand and the thermometer with the other throughout the procedure.

— The most common problem related to taking rectal temperatures is rectal perforation, which is mainly a risk for newborns and infants. Also, several cases of broken and retained rectal thermometers occur each year with children in the home. Because of this, many hospitals require axillary temperature measurements for infants and children.

— Know and follow your facility's policies for taking rectal temperatures in infants and children.

• In some facilities, tympanic temperatures are used for all patients, including infants and children. When taking a tympanic temperature on a pediatric patient:
— Position the probe so the tip points at the midpoint between the eyebrow and sideburn on the opposite side of the face.
— If the patient is a child *under age 3*, the pinna of the ear should be pulled down and back.
— If the patient is a child *over age 3*, the pinna of the ear should be pulled up and back.
— *Failure to use the ear tug means infrared thermometers are only partially directed at the tympanic membrane, increasing the likelihood of an inaccurate reading.*

• When taking complete vital signs on an infant or child, take the rectal temperature last in the sequence. Although this is not a painful procedure, checking the rectal temperature first may cause the infant to cry, which will accelerate the pulse and respirations.

• Evaluate the child by touch if you suspect he or she has a fever. Several studies have shown the touch method is accurate for determining whether fever is present in infants and children. If the child feels warm or hot to touch, obtain a thermometer and check the value.

• Parents may ask you to sponge a child to bring a fever down. Some physicians order this treatment for high fever. Nursing research has shown this method of lowering the temperature is of questionable value, and causes discomfort if a child develops "goose bumps" and shivering. Shivering is a compensatory mechanism to raise the temperature, so this is not the best method of fever management. Consult the nurse before sponging an infant or child. Never add alcohol to the water used for the sponge bath in infants and children.

• The alcohol-based glass thermometer continues to be considered the gold standard for temperature accuracy. Variable readings have been obtained with other types of thermometers. Follow your facility's policies and the nurse's instructions.

• Before taking a rectal temperature on an infant or child, be certain you are permitted to use this method. Check with the nurse, if necessary.

• Always hold the rectal thermometer in place while taking the temperature. Wear gloves and apply the principles of standard precautions. Insert the (rectal) glass thermometer:
— one-half inch (½") for newborn infants
— three-quarters inch (¾") for children to age 1
— one inch (1") for children ages 1 to 5

(continues)

Table 1-4 "BEST PRACTICES" FOR TAKING VITAL SIGNS IN INFANTS AND CHILDREN (CONTINUED)

— one to one and one-half inches (1½") for children over age 5, if necessary. Consider other methods first.

— some electronic thermometers are inserted one-fourth of an inch (¼"); follow manufacturer's instructions for the thermometer you are using.

• Studies have shown that taking the pulse and respirations for 60 seconds produces more accurate values than using 15 seconds or 30 seconds. In several studies, using a stethoscope for counting pulse and respirations also provided more accurate values. Follow facility policies for the method to use.

Vital signs is an area in which additional nursing research needs to be done. For additional information, see: Evidence Based Practice Information Sheets for Health Professionals—*Vital Signs: Best Practice,* http://www.joannabriggs.edu.au/pdf/bpvit.pdf, and Wong on the Web, http://www3.us.elsevierhealth.com/WOW/.

Table 1-5a TEMPERATURE CONVERSION FORMULAS

To convert Fahrenheit to centigrade, subtract 32 from °F, multiply by 5, and divide by 9:

$$\frac{5(°F - 32)}{9}$$

To convert centigrade to Fahrenheit, multiply °C by 9, divide by 5, and add 32:

$$\frac{°C \times 9}{5} + 32$$

Table 1-5b SIMPLIFIED FORMULAS FOR TEMPERATURE CONVERSION

TO CONVERT	TO	MULTIPLY BY
Degrees Fahrenheit	Degrees Celsius	5/9 (after subtracting 32)
Degrees Celsius	Degrees Fahrenheit	9/5 (then add 32)

PULSE

The pulse should be counted for a full 30 seconds and multiplied by two to give the beats per minute. If taking for the first time or if the pulse is irregular, it should be counted for a full minute. See Table 1-6.

Report a pulse rate that is faster or slower than normal for the patient. The normal pulse has a regular rhythm. If the rhythm is irregular, it should be reported to the nurse. The quality of the pulse should also be noted. Is it weak and thready (easily

Table 1-6   AVERAGE PULSE RATES

PATIENT	BEATS PER MINUTE
Adult men	60–70
Adult women	65–80
Children over 7 years	75–100
Preschoolers	80–110
Infants	120–160

obliterated by pressure on the pulse site) or strong and bounding (not easily obliterated by pressure)? Both are considered deviations from normal and should be reported to the nurse.

Also report:

- Pulse rates over 100 beats per minute (tachycardia)
- Pulse rates under 60 beats per minute (bradycardia)

When recording the pulse rate, it is also useful to include the position of the patient at the time of the reading because the rate can differ with postural changes.

Pulse rates can be affected by:

- Illness
- Pain
- Emotions
- Age

Table 1-7   PULSE SITES

SITE	REASON FOR USING
Radial	Readily accessible for routine use.
Temporal	Used when radial pulse is not accessible. Also easily accessed for routine evaluation of children's pulse.
Carotid	Used in emergencies because it does not require the removal of clothing. Used when peripheral pulsations cannot be felt.
	Gently rest fingers on carotid pulse. Too much pressure can impede blood flow to the brain. Caution: *Do not count both carotid pulses simultaneously*!
Apical	Used when peripheral pulse is irregular and for patients with known cardiovascular disease. Used to determine whether there is a pulse deficit (difference between apical and radial pulse).
Brachial	Used when measuring blood pressure. Used to evaluate blood flow to lower arm.
Femoral	Used to evaluate blood flow to lower limbs. Used in cases of cardiac arrest or shock.
Popliteal	Used to evaluate blood flow to lower leg.
Posterior tibial	Used to evaluate blood flow to the ankle and foot. Difficult to access in obese people or when the ankle is edematous.
Pedal	Used to evaluate blood flow to the foot and toes.

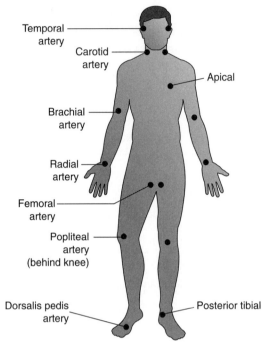

Figure 1-2A Pulse points.

- Exercise
- Elevated temperature
- Gender (slightly faster in women than in men)
- Position
- Physical training
- Lowered temperature
- Drugs

When counting a peripheral pulse to evaluate blood flow to an area of the body, the nursing assistant should also count the pulse on the other side of the body and compare them. The pulses on the lower limbs may be difficult to feel, especially in those patients who have cardiovascular problems or who have had surgery on the limbs. In these cases it is more important to note whether a pulse is absent.

When evaluating circulation to the limbs, also note such factors as the color of the area below the pulse point; whether it is hot, warm, or cold to the touch and whether the patient is able to freely move it. Report any deviation from normal to the nurse.

Refer to Figures 1-2A, B, C, and D and Table 1-7 regarding common pulse sites of the body.

RESPIRATION

Count pulse and respirations during the same procedure. Respirations should be counted immediately following the pulse count without telling the patient. The patient's hand is kept in the same position, and your fingers remain on the pulse so that you seem to still be taking the pulse. The rate and volume of respirations may change if the patient knows they are being counted.

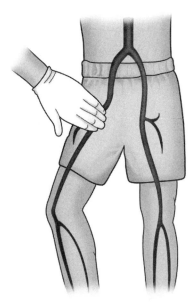

Figure 1-2B The femoral pulse is in the crease of the upper leg.

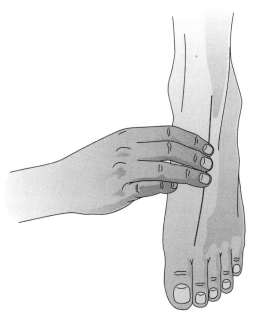

Figure 1-2C To locate the dorsalis pedis pulse, draw an imaginary line from the ankle to the area between the great toe and second toe.

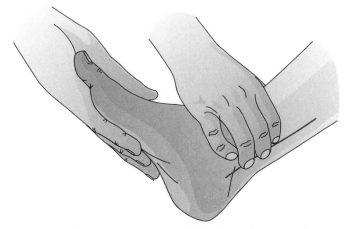

Figure 1-2D To locate the posterior tibial pulses, place your fingers in the groove between the Achilles tendon and the tibia. Move your fingers in slightly, toward the tibia.

An inspiration and expiration are counted as one respiration. Count for 30 seconds and multiply by two if the respirations are regular. Count for the full 60 seconds if they are irregular.

Factors that affect respiratory rates are similar to those listed as affecting pulse rates. See Table 1-8 for average respiratory rates.

Report any deviation in respirations from normal to the nurse.

What to Note

The rate, rhythm, symmetry, volume, and character of respirations should be noted.

The rate is normal for an adult if it is between 12 and 20 respirations per minute. Do not forget that all vital signs are compared to previous readings for that patient because they may normally deviate from the average rates.

Table 1-8   AVERAGE RESPIRATORY RATES

AGE	RESPIRATIONS PER MINUTE	AVERAGE RANGE
Newborn	35	30–60
1 year	30	24–40
2 years	28	22–34
Child	25	18–30
Adolescent	18	12–24
Adult	16	12–20
Older adult	20	15–25

- *Tachypnea* refers to rapid breathing, more than 20 breaths per minute.
- *Bradypnea* refers to slow breathing, fewer than 12 breaths per minute.
- Rhythm refers to regularity.
- *Apnea* refers to absence of respirations.
- *Cheyne-Stokes respirations* occur when there is a period of difficult or labored breathing followed by periods of apnea.
- *Symmetry* is the ability of the chest to expand equally on each side as air enters the lungs.
- *Volume* is the depth of respirations. Is the depth normal, shallow (the movement of the chest can hardly be seen), or deep (a large volume of air is exchanged with each breath)?
- *Character* refers to the aspects of the patient's respirations that are different from normal.
- *Dyspnea* is difficult or labored breathing. Note whether the patient has dyspnea after walking or if it is severe enough to prevent him or her from talking in full sentences.
- *Orthopnea* is a type of dyspnea when there is an inability to breathe unless in a seated or upright position.

Immediately report dyspnea or a patient's complaint about difficulty with breathing to the nurse. Also report noisy respirations.

- Respirations that sound like snoring are referred to as *stertorous.* These can be caused by secretions in the large airways and can be cleared by coughing. Other conditions may also cause stertorous respirations.
- *Crackles* are moist respirations. These sound like the noise made when you roll a lock of hair between your fingers near your ear. These are caused by air passing through secretions in the lower airways and usually do not clear with coughing.
- *Gurgles* are commonly heard in the dying patient and are caused by air passing through moist secretions in the respiratory tract.
- *Wheezing* is difficult breathing caused by air passing through narrowed airways.

BLOOD PRESSURE

Blood pressure is the measure of the pressure of the blood as it moves through the arteries. Blood pressure varies with contraction (systole) and relaxation (diastole) of the ventricles of the heart. The systolic reading measures the pressure when the ventricles have contracted and blood is forced out into the arteries. It is when the pressure within the arteries is greatest. The diastolic reading measures the pressure when the ventricles have relaxed. The systolic pressure is written above the diastolic pressure, for example, systolic/diastolic = 110/70. See Table 1-9.

The difference between the systolic and diastolic pressure is called the *pulse pressure.* The average pulse pressure in a healthy adult is about 40 mm Hg (range 30–50 mm Hg). An increase in blood volume or heart rate or a decrease in the ability of arteries to expand because of aging or disease can result in increased pulse pressure.

Use the correct size cuff or the BP reading will be inaccurate. The length of the cuff bladder should equal 80% of the circumference of the patient's arm. The width of the cuff should measure approximately 40% of the circumference of the patient's arm. A cuff that is too narrow will give high readings, and one that is too wide will give low readings. See Table 1-10.

Table 1-9 FACTORS AFFECTING BLOOD PRESSURE (BP)

FACTORS THAT INCREASE BP	FACTORS THAT DECREASE BP
Sex (males slightly higher)	Fasting
Exercise	Rest
Eating	Depressants
Stimulants	Weight loss
Emotional stress	Abnormal conditions such as hemorrhage (loss of blood) or shock
Disease such as arteriosclerosis, diabetes, and increased cholesterol	Some medications (such as antihypertensives, used to lower the BP, and diuretics, used to lower the volume of body fluids)
Hereditary factors	
Pain	
Obesity	
Age	
Condition of blood vessels	
Some medications	

Table 1-10 CAUSES OF INACCURATE BP READINGS

Use of a wrong size cuff

An improperly wrapped cuff

Incorrect positioning of arm

Not using the same arm for all readings

Not having the gauge at eye level

Deflating the cuff too rapidly or slowly

Mistaking an auscultatory gap (sound fades out for 10–15 mm Hg and then begins again) as the diastolic pressure

Do not attempt to measure blood pressure using an arm that is the site of an intravenous infusion, that is paralyzed or injured, that is the site of a dialysis access device, if edema is present, or if surgery has been performed on that arm or on the breast on that side.

- The BP reading should be taken with the patient's arm at chest level. If the arm is higher, the BP will be decreased. If the arm is lower, the BP will be increased.

- If you need to repeat the reading, wait 1 to 2 minutes to allow a return to normal pressure within the vessels.

- Do not take BP within 30 minutes of the patient exercising, smoking, or drinking caffeine.

- Ensure that the patient does not have a full bladder because this may elevate the reading.

Report any deviations from the patient's normal readings to the nurse.

Table 1-11 BLOOD PRESSURE VARIATION ACCORDING TO AGE	
AGE	AVERAGE BP (mm Hg)
Newborn	80/45
1 year	90/60
6 years	100/65
10 years	110/70
14–adult	120/80
Older adult	140/90

- Hypertension (high blood pressure) is when values are greater than 140 mm Hg systolic and 90 mm Hg diastolic.
- Hypotension (low blood pressure) is when values in an adult are lower than 100 mm Hg systolic and 60 mm Hg diastolic. Excessive hypotension can lead to shock.

See Table 1-11.

Postural Hypotension

Sometimes you might be asked to evaluate a patient for orthostatic or postural hypotension, which is the dropping of BP when the patient moves from a sitting position to a standing position. This can cause the patient to become dizzy, light-headed, or faint. A drop in systolic pressure of 15 mm Hg or more, in diastolic of 10 mm Hg or more, and an increase in heart rate of more than 20 beats per minute is significant and should be reported to the nurse. Wait 1 to 3 minutes after the patient changes position before taking the measurement.

Note the following:

- If you were unable to hear the reading.
- If blood pressure is higher or lower than previous readings.

- If the site of the reading was other than the brachial artery.

If you cannot hear the pulse or palpate (take the measurement by feeling for the appearance and disappearance of the pulse), try on a different limb.

BLOOD PRESSURE GUIDELINES FOR ADULTS 18 OR OVER

High blood pressure, or hypertension, is the most significant risk factor for stroke and heart failure and a leading risk factor for heart disease. Having high blood pressure over a period of time increases the risk of kidney damage. Unfortunately, approximately 50 million adults (1 in 4 adults) in the United States have hypertension, but many are not aware of it. High blood pressure is called a "silent killer" because it has no signs or symptoms. Preventing high blood pressure reduces the risk of serious complications. If you have hypertension, adopting a healthy lifestyle today helps reduce the risk.

Clinical Practice Guidelines

In 2003, the National Heart, Lung, and Blood Institute (NHLBI) released new clinical practice guidelines for the prevention, detection, and treatment

Table 1-12   NATIONAL HEART, LUNG, AND BLOOD INSTITUTE BLOOD PRESSURE DEFINITIONS 2003

	BLOOD PRESSURE LEVEL (mm Hg)		
Category	Systolic	*	Diastolic
Normal	<120	and	<80
Prehypertension	120–139	or	80–89
HIGH BLOOD PRESSURE			
Stage I Hypertension	140–159	or	90–99
Stage II Hypertension	≥160	or	≥100

Legend
< means less than
≥ means greater than or equal to
Source: National Heart, Lung, and Blood Institute
National Institutes of Health 2003
For additional information, see http://www.nhlbi.nih.gov/hbp/index.html

of high blood pressure. These guidelines include a new *prehypertension* category. Having a blood pressure value between 120/80 mm Hg and 139/89 mm Hg qualifies the person for the *prehypertension* category. Although the person does not have high blood pressure now, he or she is likely to develop it in the future. About two-thirds of people over age 65 have high blood pressure.

Interpreting Blood Pressure Values

Both numbers in the blood pressure are important. In persons age 50 or over, the *systolic blood pressure value gives the most accurate diagnosis of high blood pressure.* A person with a blood pressure of 140 mm Hg systolic or above (in two or more readings) qualifies for a diagnosis of hypertension. A single high reading is not enough to make a hypertension diagnosis.

Blood Pressure Categories

The 2003 Clinical Practice Guidelines use the values in Table 1-12 to evaluate the blood pressure and risk factors.

The goal of treatment is to reduce blood pressure to less than 140 mm Hg systolic and less than 90 mm Hg diastolic. For individuals with diabetes and chronic kidney disease, the goal is to reduce blood pressure to less than 130 systolic and less than 80 diastolic.

VITAL SIGN OBSERVATIONS

An overview of vital sign observations to make and report is listed in Table 1-13.

Table 1-13   OBSERVATIONS TO MAKE AND REPORT RELATED TO THE VITAL SIGNS

- Pulse rate below 60 or above 100
- Pulse irregular, weak, or bounding
- Blood pressure below 100/60 or above 140/90
- Unable to hear blood pressure or palpate pulse
- Pain over center, left, or right chest
- Chest pain that radiates to shoulder, neck, jaw, or arm
- Shortness of breath, dyspnea, or any abnormal respirations
- Headache, dizziness, weakness, paralysis, vomiting
- Cold, blue, or gray appearance
- Cold, blue, numb, painful feet or hands
- Feeling faint or lightheaded, losing consciousness

- Respiratory rate below 12 or above 20
- Irregular respirations
- Noisy, labored respirations
- Dyspnea
- Shortness of breath
- Gasping for breath
- Cheyne-Stokes respirations
- Wheezing
- Coughing (dry or moist/productive)
- Retractions
- Using accessory muscles in the neck, chest, and/or abdomen during respiration
- Blue color of lips or nail beds, mucous membranes

- Change in weight of 5 or more pounds (increase or decrease) compared with previous weight, or according to the care plan and nurses' instructions.

OBSERVATIONS

OBSERVATIONAL SKILLS

An important nursing skill is the ability to observe the patient and report your findings. To be able to do this, you need to have a knowledge of what is normal for that person and what is usual for his or her age-group. This will allow you to recognize deviations from normal. The observations you collect will be based on your interaction with the patient, your use of equipment such as a thermometer, and your senses of sight, smell, hearing, and touch. To make accurate observations it is helpful to approach your data collection in a systematic way, taking note of the following.

Circulatory System

- Pulse—strength, regularity, rate, skipped beats
- Blood pressure (sitting and standing)

Integumentary System

- Color—flushed, pink, pale, red, jaundiced, mottled, cyanotic (bluish)
- Temperature—warm, hot, cool
- Moisture—dry, moist, perspiring
- Nails—pale, pink, or cyanotic
- Abnormalities—rashes, bruises, scars, pressure ulcers, areas of redness, bleeding, edema, dryness, masses, odors, itching, dandruff, psoriasis, moles

Musculoskeletal System

- Activity level—actual, range of motion of all joints, fatigue
- Posture—stooped, curled up in bed, straight
- Mobility—ability to move in bed, to get out of bed, to stand, to walk, and to maintain balance
- Joints—deformities, stiffness, masses, swelling, pain, tenderness
- Muscles—paralysis, weakness, cramps, spasms, rigidity, tremors

Respiratory System

- Respirations (breathing)—rate, regularity, depth, difficulty in breathing, shortness of breath with exertion or when still, wheezing or crackling heard, breathing through nose or mouth
- Cough—frequency, dry, loose, productive
- Color and consistency of any sputum

Urinary System

- Urination—frequency, amount, color, clarity, odor, urgency, burning, pain, dribbling, presence of blood or sediment, ability to hold urine, incontinence, urination at night

Digestive System

- Appetite—amount of fluid and food consumed, tolerance to food, belching or burping

- Eating—difficulty chewing or swallowing
- Nausea and/or vomiting, indigestion
- Bowel elimination—frequency, amount, consistency, color of stools, diarrhea, constipation, incontinence, flatus, difficulty in passing stool
- Mouth—odor, pain, ability to speak, taste, ulcers, burning, coating, color of gums, bleeding, absence of teeth, cavities, voice change, dentures
- Abdomen—size, fat, muscle tone, distension, abnormal pulsations, sounds (absent), tenderness, rigidity, pain
- Rectum—hemorrhoids, excoriation, rashes, abscess, masses, tenderness, pain, itching, burning

Endocrine System

- Signs and symptoms of diabetes (hypoglycemia, hyperglycemia), blood sugar

Nervous System

- Mental status—conscious, orientation to time, place, person
- Ability to make verbal or nonverbal responses
- Attitude—cooperative, negative, hostile, withdrawn
- Mood—happy, sad, flat
- Speech—loud, clear, hoarse, quick, coherent, vague, logical, confused

Reproductive System

Female

- Breasts—color of nipples, presence of lumps, discolorations, dimpling, swelling, discharge, inversion, pain, symmetry
- Menstrual periods—frequency, amount and character of bleeding, cramping, excessive bleeding
- Vaginal drainage—amount, odor, and character

- Genitals—swelling, ulcerations, masses, tenderness, pain

Male

- Testes—lumps, size, shape, swelling, absence
- Penis—amount and color of drainage, ulceration, pain

Senses

- Eyes—reddened, yellow, color of drainage, pupils equal in size, pain, burning, sensitivity to light
- Ears—drainage, difficulty hearing, pain, ringing, hearing noises, dizziness
- Nose—color of drainage, bleeding, loss of sense of smell, pain, tenderness
- Sense of touch—ability to feel pressure and pain
- Taste—metallic taste, unusual tastes, loss of sense of taste

Other Observations

In addition to observations about body systems, you will also need to note facts related to pain, behavior, and ability to perform activities of daily living.

Pain—location; type of pain (sharp, dull, aching, churning, throbbing); does it radiate to anywhere; constant or intermittent or related to specific activities; time pain started; if medication was given, did it relieve the pain; can the person sleep with the pain; posture; facial expression; is it similar to pain he or she has experienced previously?

Behavior—anxious, phobic, confused, agitated, uncooperative, hostile, passive, withdrawn, overactive, underactive, assaultive, violent, irritable, excitable, compulsive movements.

Activities of daily living—ability to carry out activities, assistance required, use of adaptive devices, eating without assistance, requires assistance eating, meals cut up, food mechanically altered, positioning for eating, ability to shower and bathe, combing and brushing hair, brushing teeth, ability to use bathroom, ability to dress, ability to get out of bed and in and out of chair, ability to walk.

Observations must be:

- Accurate and timely.
- Reported to the nurse immediately if unusual for the patient.
- Documented in the patient's record, either by you or by the nurse.

Reporting Normal Observations

Sometimes you may be expected to report "normal" observations. This information tells the nurse and physician whether the patient's condition is improving. For example, if a patient has had a respiratory tract infection and the signs and symptoms have diminished, it is important to report "no coughing or respiratory distress is noted." See Tables 2-1 through 2-9 for signs and symptoms of illness.

Table 2-1 GENERAL OBSERVATION AND REPORTING GUIDELINES

GENERAL SIGNS AND SYMPTOMS OF ILLNESS THAT SHOULD BE REPORTED TO THE NURSE IMMEDIATELY

Chest pain
Shortness of breath
Difficulty breathing
Weakness or dizziness
Headache
Pain, facial expressions or body language suggesting pain
Nausea or vomiting
Diarrhea (multiple loose stools; one loose stool is not diarrhea)
Cough
Cyanosis or change in color
Change in mental status
Excessive thirst
Lethargy
Unusual drainage from a wound or body cavity
Abnormal appearance of urine or feces
Unable to hear blood pressure or palpate pulse
Changes in vital signs
Abnormal behavior, including crying
Requests for medication for an acute problem

Table 2-2   SPECIFIC OBSERVATION AND REPORTING GUIDELINES

SYSTEM OR PROBLEM	OBSERVATION TO REPORT
Evidence of pain	Chest pain
	Pain that radiates
	Pain upon movement
	Pain during urination
	Pain when having a bowel movement
	Splinting an area upon movement
	Grimacing, or facial expressions suggesting pain
	Body language suggesting pain
	Unrelieved pain after pain medication has been given
	Pain is *never* normal; *all* complaints of pain should be reported to the nurse promptly.
Cardiovascular system	Abnormal pulse below 60 or above 100
	Pulse irregular, weak, or bounding
	Change in pulse strength, regularity, rate, skipped beats
	Blood pressure below 100/60 or above 140/90 mm Hg
	Unable to hear blood pressure or palpate pulse
	Pain over center, left, or right chest
	Chest pain that radiates to shoulder, neck, jaw, or arm
	Shortness of breath, dyspnea, or any abnormal respirations
	Headache, dizziness, weakness, paralysis, vomiting
	Cold, blue, or gray appearance
	Cold, blue, numb, painful feet or hands
	Capillary refill >3 seconds
Respiratory system	Respiratory rate below 12 or above 20
	Irregular respirations
	Noisy, labored respirations
	Dyspnea
	Shortness of breath
	Shortness of breath upon exertion
	Gasping for breath
	Cheyne-Stokes respirations
	Wheezing or crackling
	New-onset breathing through mouth
	Coughing (dry or moist/productive)
	Retractions
	Blue color of lips or nail beds, mucous membranes
	Capillary refill >3 seconds
	Pulse oximeter <90%

(continues)

Table 2-2 SPECIFIC OBSERVATION AND REPORTING GUIDELINES (CONTINUED)

SYSTEM OR PROBLEM	OBSERVATION TO REPORT
Integumentary system	Rash
	Redness
	Redness in the skin that does not go away within 30 minutes after pressure is relieved from a bony prominence or pressure area
	In dark- or yellow-skinned patients, spots or areas that are darker in appearance than normal skin tone
	Pressure ulcers
	Irritation
	Bruises
	Skin discoloration
	Swelling
	Lumps
	Abnormal skin growths
	Moles or warts
	Change in color of a wart or mole
	Abnormal sweating
	Excessive heat or coolness to touch
	Open areas/skin breakdown
	Drainage
	Foul odor
	Complaints such as numbness, burning, tingling, itching
	Signs of infection
	Cyanosis or unusual skin color, such as blue or gray color of the skin, lips, nail beds, roof of mouth, or mucous membranes
	Other abnormal color of skin, including flushed, pink, pale, jaundiced, mottled
	Skin growths
	Poor skin turgor/tenting of skin on forehead or over sternum
	Sunken, dark eyes
	Itching or scratching
	Bleeding
	Excessive dryness
	Masses
	Odors
	Dandruff, psoriasis
Gastrointestinal system	Sores or ulcers inside the mouth
	Difficulty chewing or swallowing food

Table 2-2   SPECIFIC OBSERVATION AND REPORTING GUIDELINES (CONTINUED)

SYSTEM OR PROBLEM	OBSERVATION TO REPORT
	Unusual or abnormal appearance of feces
	Blood, mucus, parasites, or other unusual substances in stool
	Unusual color of feces
	Hard stool, difficulty passing stool
	Extremely small or extremely large stool
	Loose, watery stool
	Unusual color stool
	Complaints of pain, constipation, diarrhea, bleeding
	Frequent belching
	Changes in appetite
	Excessive thirst
	Fruity smell to breath
	Complaints of indigestion
	Excessive gas (flatus)
	Nausea, vomiting
	Difficulty chewing or swallowing
	Choking
	Abdominal pain
	Abdominal distention (swelling)
	Oral or rectal bleeding
	Vomitus, stool, or drainage from a nasogastric tube that looks like coffee grounds
	Mouth odor, pain, ability to speak, taste, ulcers, burning, coating, color of gums, bleeding, absence of teeth, cavities, voice change, dentures
	Change in abdomen size, muscle tone, abnormal pulsations, tenderness, rigidity, pain
	Rectal hemorrhoids, masses, tenderness, pain, itching, burning
Nutritional problems	Increase or decrease in food (caloric) intake
	Increase or decrease of body weight
	Diabetic patients who do not eat all their food or who eat more than allowed on diet
	Patients on restricted diets who do not adhere to their diet
	Refusal to accept meal, supplement, snack
	Refusal to accept food substitute for meat or vegetable
	Meal intake of less than 50% (or 75%, according to facility policy)

(continues)

Table 2-2 SPECIFIC OBSERVATION AND REPORTING GUIDELINES (CONTINUED)

SYSTEM OR PROBLEM	OBSERVATION TO REPORT
Genitourinary system	Urinary output too low
	Oral intake too low
	Urinary output greatly exceeds fluid intake
	Fluid intake and output not reasonably balanced
	Abnormal appearance of urine: dark, concentrated, red, cloudy
	Unusual substances in urine: blood, pus, particles, sediment
	Complaints of difficulty urinating
	Foul-smelling urine
	Complaints of pain, burning, urgency, frequency, pain in lower back
	Urinating frequently in small amounts
	Sudden-onset incontinence
	Edema; obvious fluid in tissues, particularly face, fingers, legs, ankles, feet
	Sudden weight loss or gain
	Respiratory distress
	Changes in mental status
	Patient complains of inability to empty bladder or cannot empty bladder completely
	Changes from normal for patient, including frequency, amount, color, clarity, odor, urgency, dribbling, incontinence, urination during the night
Reproductive system, female	Breasts—color of nipples
	Presence of lumps
	Discolorations
	Localized pain or tenderness
	Dimpling
	Swelling
	Discharge
	Inversion
	Symmetry
	Menstrual periods—frequency, amount and character of bleeding, cramping, excessive bleeding
	Vaginal drainage—amount, odor, character
	External genitals—swelling, ulcerations, masses, tenderness, pain
Reproductive system, male	Testes—lumps, size, shape, swelling, absence
	Penis—amount and color of drainage, ulceration, pain

Table 2-2   SPECIFIC OBSERVATION AND REPORTING GUIDELINES (CONTINUED)

SYSTEM OR PROBLEM	OBSERVATION TO REPORT
Fluid balance problems	Fluid intake or output too high
	Fluid intake or output too low
	Patients with fluid restrictions exceeding limitations
	Fluid intake and output not reasonably balanced
	Signs of dehydration, including low fluid intake, low output of dark urine with strong odor, weight loss, dry skin, dry mucous membranes of the lips, mouth, tongue, eyes, drowsiness, confusion
Furrows or lines in tongue	Patients who are mouth breathers may appear to have very dry mucous membranes. The area between the gums and cheek will stay moist, however, *unless the patient is dehydrated.*
	Edema—obvious fluid in tissues, particularly face, fingers, legs, ankles, feet
Nervous system	Change in level of consciousness, orientation, awareness, or alertness
	New onset of inability to recognize familiar persons or objects
	New onset of disorientation; does not know person, place, time
	Increasing memory or mental confusion, worsening confusion
	Progressive lethargy
	Loss of sensation
	Numbness, tingling
	Change in pupil size, unequal pupils
	Abnormal or involuntary motor function
	Spasticity
	Loss of ability to move a body part
	Incoordination
	Changes in speech
	Changes in ability to swallow
	Drooping of one side of the face
	New onset of weakness or paralysis on one side of the body
Musculoskeletal system	Pain
	Deformity
	Stiffness, swelling, pain, tenderness in joints
	Edema
	Immobility

(continues)

Table 2-2   SPECIFIC OBSERVATION AND REPORTING GUIDELINES (CONTINUED)

SYSTEM OR PROBLEM	OBSERVATION TO REPORT
	Inability to move arms and legs
	Inability to move one or more joints
	Limited or abnormal range of motion
	New onset of fatigue
	Shortening and external rotation of one leg in patient with history of falls
	Sudden onset of falls, difficulty balancing
	Jerking, tremors, shaky movements, rigidity, muscle spasms
	Weakness
	Sensory changes
	Change in ability to sit, stand, move, or walk
	Change in ability to balance
	Pain upon movement
	Change in posture—stooped, curled up in bed, straight
Mental status	Change in consciousness, awareness, or alertness
	Change in mood, behavior, or emotional status
	Change in orientation to person, place, time, season
	Change in communication
	Change in memory
	Excessive drowsiness
	Change in ability to respond verbally or nonverbally
	Sleepiness for no apparent reason
	Sudden onset of mental confusion
	Threats of suicide or harm to self or others
	Attitude—cooperative, negative, hostile, withdrawn
	Mood—happy, sad, flat
	Speech—loud, clear, hoarse, quick, coherent, vague, logical, confused, slurred
Senses	Eyes—reddened, yellow, drainage, color of drainage, pupils equal in size, pain, burning, sensitivity to light
	Ears—drainage, difficulty hearing, pain, ringing, hearing noises, dizziness
	Nose—color of drainage, bleeding, loss of sense of smell, pain, tenderness
	Sense of touch—ability to feel heat and cold, pressure, pain, presence of numbness or tingling
	Taste—metallic, unusual, loss of sense of taste

Table 2-3   IMPORTANT OBSERVATIONS OF DIABETIC PATIENTS

Inadequate food intake
Eating food not permitted on diet
Refusal of meals, supplements, or snacks
Nausea, vomiting, or diarrhea
Inadequate fluid intake
Excessive activity
Complaints of dizziness, shakiness, racing heart
Blood sugar values outside of normal range

SIGNS AND SYMPTOMS OF HYPERGLYCEMIA	SIGNS AND SYMPTOMS OF HYPOGLYCEMIA
Nausea, vomiting	Complaints of hunger, weakness, dizziness, shakiness
Weakness	
Headache	Skin cold, moist, clammy, pale
Full, bounding pulse	Rapid, shallow respirations
Fruity smell to breath	Nervousness and excitement
Hot, dry, flushed skin	Rapid pulse
Labored respirations	Unconsciousness
Drowsiness	No sugar in the urine
Mental confusion	Low blood sugar by finger stick
Unconsciousness	
Sugar in the urine	
High blood sugar by finger stick	

Table 2-4   OBSERVATIONS RELATED TO BREATHING

MONITORING FOR BREATHING ADEQUACY

Patient is talking, respirations are between 12 and 20, and there is no apparent distress.

The rhythm is regular.

Patient's color is normal, with no cyanosis or gray coloration.

Look at the patient's chest. It should expand equally with each inspiration.

Listen for breath sounds by placing your ear next to the patient's nose and mouth, if necessary. The sounds should be quiet, without gurgling, wheezing, gasping, or other abnormal sounds.

Feel for breath movement on your cheek and ear.

Capillary refill <3 seconds.

Pulse oximeter exceeds 95%.

Table 2-5 OBSERVATIONS RELATED TO INADEQUATE OXYGENATION

SIGNS AND SYMPTOMS OF DECREASED OXYGENATION

Unusual skin color, such as dusky, pale, blue, or gray

Unusual color of the lips, mucous membranes, nail beds, lining or roof of mouth

Capillary refill >3 seconds

Pulse oximeter <90%

Cool, clammy skin

Slow, rapid, or irregular breathing

Shortness of breath or difficulty breathing

Noisy breathing

Gasping for breath

Changes in mental status, including decreased responsiveness, drowsiness, sleepiness for no apparent reason, restlessness, becomes more confused

Tachycardia

Table 2-6 OBSERVATIONS RELATED TO INADEQUATE BREATHING

SIGNS AND SYMPTOMS OF INADEQUATE BREATHING TO REPORT TO THE NURSE IMMEDIATELY

Movement in the chest is absent, minimal, or irregular.

Breathing movement appears to be in the abdomen, not the lungs.

Air movement cannot be detected by listening and feeling for breath sounds on your cheek and ear.

Respiratory rate is too slow or rapid.

Respirations are irregular, gasping, very deep, or shallow.

Respirations appear labored.

Patient is short of breath.

Patient's skin, lips, tongue, earlobes, mucous membranes, or nail beds are blue or gray.

Patient is unable to speak at all or cannot speak in sentences because he or she is short of breath.

Respirations are noisy.

Nasal flaring is present during inspiration.

The muscles below the ribs and/or above the clavicles retract inward during respiration.

Table 2-7   PULSE OXIMETER VALUES

PULSE OXIMETER READING	INTERPRETATION	NURSING ASSISTANT ACTION
95% to 100%	Normal	No action necessary
Below 90%	Suggests complications, impending hypoxemia	Check capillary refill Report to nurse promptly
85% or below	Inadequate oxygen for body function, condition worsening, potential impending crisis	Report to nurse immediately
Below 70%	Life threatening	Stay with the patient. Use the call signal or phone to summon the nurse to the room immediately

Table 2-8   GENERAL SIGNS AND SYMPTOMS OF INFECTION

SYSTEM OR PROBLEM	OBSERVATION TO REPORT
General signs/symptoms of infection	Elevated temperature
	Hypothermia, or temperature below normal for patient
	Rapid pulse
	Rapid respirations
	Hypotension
	Fatigue
	New onset of mental confusion
	Sweating
	Chills
	Skin hot or cold to touch
	Skin flushed, red, gray, or blue
	Inflammation of skin as evidenced by redness, edema, heat, or pain
	Abnormal drainage from any part of the body
Respiratory system infection	Rapid respirations
	Irregular respirations
	Noisy, labored respirations
	Dyspnea
	Coughing
	Blue color of lips or nail beds, mucous membranes

(continues)

Table 2-8   GENERAL SIGNS AND SYMPTOMS OF INFECTION (CONTINUED)

SYSTEM OR PROBLEM	OBSERVATION TO REPORT
Integumentary system infection	Rash Redness Swelling Open areas/skin breakdown Drainage Foul odor
Gastrointestinal system infection	Unusual or abnormal appearance or color of bowel movement Blood, mucus, or other unusual substances in stool Diarrhea Complaints of indigestion or excessive gas Nausea, vomiting Abdominal pain
Genitourinary system infection	Urinary output too low Oral intake too low Abnormal appearance of urine: dark, concentrated, red, cloudy Unusual material in urine: blood, pus, particles Complaints of pain, burning, urgency, frequency, pain in lower back Edema Sudden weight loss or gain Respiratory distress Change in mental status
Mental status problems	Change in level of consciousness, awareness, or alertness Changes in mood or behavior Change in ability to express self or communicate Mental confusion

Table 2-9   WOUND OBSERVATIONS

WOUND OBSERVATIONS TO REPORT TO THE NURSE

Redness
Drainage, particularly if purulent (puslike) or foul-smelling
Heat
Edema
Increased pain or tenderness
Fever
Edema of tissue surrounding the wound
Separation of wound edges
Trauma or injury
Maceration, or a waterlogged appearance of the wound edges
Bruising
Frank bleeding

WRITING AND TALKING ABOUT IT

HEALTH INSURANCE PORTABILITY AND ACCOUNTABILITY ACT (HIPAA)

Each patient has a right to privacy with regard to his or her medical information, including information on the medical record. All staff are responsible for protecting patient information and data from access by unauthorized persons. Medical records and other patient data should be accessed only by those with a need to know the information. Staff should not read patient charts to satisfy their curiosity.

In 1996, Congress passed the *Health Insurance Portability and Accountability Act (HIPAA)*. The HIPAA rules protect all individually identifiable health information in any form. The rules apply to paper, verbal, and electronic documentation, billing records, and clinical records. Because of this, patient information is provided to staff on a "need to know" basis. In other words, information is disclosed only if staff needs it to carry out their duties. This law has many provisions. One portion applies to privacy, confidentiality, and medical records. The HIPAA rules:

- increase patient control over personal medical records.

- restrict the use and disclosure of patient information.
- make facilities accountable for protecting patient data.
- require the facility to implement and monitor their information release policies and procedures.

Facilities must monitor how and where they use patient information. Policies must protect patient charts, conversations and reports about patient information, faxing patient documents, and disclosing other personal information. Staff may not disclose names of patients on their unit when responding to telephone inquiries, and the complete names of patients are not posted where they are visible to the public. The HIPAA policies and procedures are individualized to facility operations and needs.

CHARTING

Charting should note the time the entry was made and describe your observations; describe any interventions you have used, their effectiveness, and the patient's response. Indicate the progress the patient is making toward meeting care plan goals. Refer to Tables 3-1 and 3-2.

Table 3-1 CHARTING RULES

Check for right patient, right chart, right room.

Fill out new headings completely.

Make sure the patient's name appears on each form.

Use correct color of ink (black).

Date and time each entry.

Chart entries in correct sequence.

Document on the correct form.

Make entries brief, objective (record only what has been observed), and accurate.

Do not record opinions.

Use the patient's words in quotation marks when these are of significance.

Print or write clearly.

Spell each word correctly.

Use only abbreviations that are approved by your facility.

If care was withheld for a specific reason, initial the box, circle your initials, and then explain why care was withheld in a narrative note or in the exceptions box on the back of the flow sheet.

Read what you are documenting on flow sheets. It is easy to skip up or down a line. Be sure you are documenting on the correct line.

Make sure the intake and output totals are accurate and recorded. If the fluid intake appears inadequate or intake and output do not reasonably balance, notify the nurse.

Make sure the information you are documenting is complete and accurate. If information is missing or inaccurate, notify the nurse.

Always chart after performing the procedure, never in advance.

Notify the nurse if something is missing from a computerized flow sheet. The nurse will add missing information that is listed on the patient's care plan or critical pathway. For example, your facility routinely charts that patients are turned and repositioned every 2 hours. You routinely turn and reposition Mrs. Long, according to her critical pathway. However, there is no place to document this important care on the flow sheet.

Initial for the right procedure, on the right day, on the right shift.

Your complete signature must be on each flow sheet, usually at the bottom of the page.

Remember that flow sheets are legal records.

If you forget to chart something, follow your facility policy for making a late entry note on the chart.

Table 3-2 THE 24-HOUR CLOCK

STANDARD CLOCK	24-HOUR CLOCK	STANDARD CLOCK	24-HOUR CLOCK
12:00 midnight	2400 or 0000	12:00 noon	1200
1:00 a.m.	0100	1:00 p.m.	1300
2:00 a.m.	0200	2:00 p.m.	1400
3:00 a.m.	0300	3:00 p.m.	1500
4:00 a.m.	0400	4:00 p.m.	1600
5:00 a.m.	0500	5:00 p.m.	1700
6:00 a.m.	0600	6:00 p.m.	1800
7:00 a.m.	0700	7:00 p.m.	1900
8:00 a.m.	0800	8:00 p.m.	2000
9:00 a.m.	0900	9:00 p.m.	2100
10:00 a.m.	1000	10:00 p.m.	2200
11:00 a.m.	1100	11:00 p.m.	2300

Entries in the chart are made in chronological order, by date and time. Some facilities use the 24-hour clock to document the time. When this system is used, indicating times by noting a.m. or p.m. is not necessary.

REPORTING

An oral report is used to relay information to the nurse or other assistants. Reports should:

- Be brief.
- Be prompt.
- Be accurate.
- Be objective.
- State patient's name, room, and bed number.
- State what was unusual or abnormal and the time the observations were made. This includes changes in the patient's routine.
- Include activities that were not completed on your shift.
- Include changes to the patient's care.

If you are relaying something the patient has told you, because it is pertinent to his or her care, repeat it exactly the way the patient said it.

Examples:

- Mr. Jones in 249 says it hurts every time he urinates.
- Mrs. Goldberg was wandering around the hall and said she did not know where she was.

To report other observations, state your measurements or facts.

Examples:

- Mrs. Dominick's blood pressure is 142/86 mm Hg.
- Mr. Hernandez ate only 50% of his meal at lunchtime.
- Mrs. Hughes is crying.

If you are reporting a patient's symptom, it is better to provide extra information. For example, if the patient has pain:

- Describe the pain, when it started, where it is located, and how severe the patient says it is.

- Did the patient state the pain was brought on by anything in particular?
- Are any other symptoms associated with the pain, such as nausea?

Hand-Off Communication

Hand-off communication is essential communication that must occur when a patient transfers care from one worker or department to another worker or department. This is a very vulnerable time for the patient and is one of the most likely times for errors to occur. Information included in the hand-off report should include a brief summary of the patient's:

- situation and background.
- relevant problems, observations, and findings.
- recommendations for continuity of ongoing care.

Hand-off communication must be accurate, clear, and complete. It should also include an opportunity to ask questions. As a nursing assistant, you will be giving and receiving hand-off information. Write down information about your patients, if necessary, and refer to your notes to make sure all of the elements listed here are met when providing hand-off reports.

End-of-Duty Report

When you report off duty at the end of the shift, report to the nurse:

- The condition of each of the patients you were assigned to
- The care you gave each patient
- Observations you made while giving care

SHIFT REPORTS

Shift reports are used to communicate information about patients. The report will include:

- Changes in patients' conditions
- Information about new patients
- Names of patients who were discharged or died
- Any incidents that occurred to patients
- New physicians' orders
- Special events for the patients that will occur during your shift

The report will help you plan your assignment. Your assignment tells you:

- Which patients you will care for during your shift
- The procedures you will need to do for these patients

Your supervising nurse will then give you additional information about your assignment based on the shift report. This information may include orders to complete procedures for specific patients:

- Take temperature, pulse, respirations, blood pressure, and weights on designated patients.
- Allow a patient to remain in bed because of a change in condition.
- Make observations of a patient who has had a recent change of condition. See Table 3-3 for reporting guidelines.
- Special patient needs, schedules, or things to watch for.

Table 3-3   REPORTING GUIDELINES

In general, you should report:

Changes in the patient's mood, behavior, or mental status.

Changes in the patient's vital signs.

Comments or complaints the patient makes about his or her condition, such as pain, dizziness, numbness, and so forth.

Patient complaints.

Changes in the patient's body that you can see.

What you observe using your senses of hearing, touch, smell, and sight.

Care that works well for the patient.

Approaches that are not working for the patient.

If you report observations to the nurse and the patient's condition seems to worsen, inform the nurse again.

GETTING THINGS DONE

TIME MANAGEMENT: A KEY TO NURSING ASSISTANT SUCCESS

Successful time management is a key to nursing assistant success. Time cannot be managed in the same manner as other resources. This is because time is always a borrowed commodity. Once time is used, it is gone forever and cannot be replaced. Figure 4-1 shows a breakdown of your time.

You cannot control the total amount of time available to get your work done, and you have a given amount of time in which to do your work each day. This daily allotment cannot be changed. However, you have a high degree of control over how the available time is used. Successful nursing assistants know that they can manage themselves only in relation to time. When you master good organization and time-management skills, your patients will be satisfied and you may find that other workers are emulating you and following your positive example.

TIME MANAGEMENT AND THE NURSING PROCESS

Nurses have many acronyms that are used for patient assessment, care, and unit management. APIE is an acronym that describes the nursing care process:

A = Assessment
P = Plan
I = Implementation
E = Evaluation

Using APIE will help you perfect your organization and time management skills. You should:

- **Assess** (evaluate) your time management problems.
- Develop a **plan** to improve your skills.
- **Implement** your plan.
- **Evaluate** and monitor the results regularly to see if your plan is working or can be improved. As working conditions, patients, and

---

1 day = 86,400 seconds or 1,440 minutes or 24 hours

1 week = 168 hours

If you work an 8-hour shift, you have:

28,800 seconds or 480 minutes in which to get your work done

If you work a 12-hour shift, you have:

43,200 seconds or 600 minutes in which to get your work done

Figure 4-1 Breakdown of Time.

situations change, you may need to further modify your plan.

—Tweak and modify your plan, if needed, and make adjustments to stay on track.

—Challenge yourself to improve upon good results.

Organizing Your Work

Time management is a tool that can help you, but only if you are realistic in organizing your time. Never take shortcuts that sacrifice safety or breach infection control practices to save time. In the long run, breaches of this nature cause problems that are more time consuming, such as if a patient falls and is injured, or if you or a patient become ill from inadequate infection control practices. Another area in which you should not cut corners is patient rights. Knocking on doors, draping patients with bath blankets during procedures, and closing the privacy curtains all take time. However, this is time well spent, and supporting patient rights shows respect for the patients and enhances patient satisfaction with care. As you gain experience, you will learn ways to safely save time without compromising patient care.

Practice organizing your work. Good organization reduces stress. Organization is not something that can be taught in the classroom. Although you have learned the basic principles in class, it is up to you to practice and master them. Organizing your work involves setting *priorities*. This includes:

* organizing and performing tasks in order of importance.
* anticipating your own supply needs and patients' personal needs.
* bringing necessary items to the room before beginning care so you

will not have to waste time and energy retrieving forgotten items.

Set priorities at the beginning of your shift to make the most of your day. This means identifying what must be done and rating each task in order of importance. Priorities continually change because of patient illness, admissions, discharges, and emergencies. Do not allow yourself to become frustrated if your priorities change or must be adjusted part way through the shift. Keep your cool, readjust your plan, and continue your work.

After you have identified your priorities, plan for the most efficient use of your time. Identify tasks that can be grouped together. For example, you can make the bed while the patient is sitting in a chair or washing at the sink. Plan your schedule around meal times, activities, appointments, and the patients' therapy schedules. Identify and plan for tasks that will require someone else to help you or for which you will need special equipment. If organization or time management are problems for you, ask other workers for tips and techniques to use.

Making Rounds

Making rounds is an important part of your time management strategy, and keeps you apprised of your patients' needs. Over the long run, you will find that it saves you many trips up and down the hallway, and gives you a more complete picture of patient needs and activities. You will find you are thinking on your feet and formulating plans for patient care as you make rounds and monitor your patients' needs.

Check on all of your patients before beginning your assignment. Take care of their immediate needs. List special procedures that must be done and the time. Check to see if patients are scheduled for tests, appointments, or other activities during your shift. Follow your assignment sheet and each patient's care plan.

Time management needs frequent evaluation and adjustment, especially if you have a day or two when your schedule goes completely off track. This sometimes happens because of situations beyond your control. Avoid becoming upset if this happens, and strive to keep your balance even. This takes some practice, but this skill can be mastered if you work hard and focus on it.

Nursing assistants sometimes wonder how to get various assigned tasks done. Consider different solutions, such as working smarter instead of harder. Try to shift your focus from the many small, individual "tasks" you do each day. Instead, look for the big picture in your responsibilities, such as:

• the importance of the observations you make in the course of caring for patients and making rounds on your assigned group.

• meeting patient needs, providing quality care, including finding time to do important little things that are meaningful to patients, and ensuring patient satisfaction.

• communicating with patients, families, and other workers.

• keeping the nurse apprised of changes in patient conditions and other important details and observations.

Those are the important part of your job, and you do them while you are simultaneously performing the many tasks you may consider tedious. Multitasking is a form of juggling your work, and you will become proficient

at it as you gain experience and work on your organizational skills. Being a nursing assistant is an important position that involves much more than performing a defined series of menial *tasks*. You are the eyes and ears of the nurses, and make a difference in the quality of care the patients receive. Your responsibilities include important skills, such as making accurate observations during the course of patient care, and using good clinical judgment when giving care and in reporting information to the nurse. To be successful, you must make good use of your time. Some benefits of effective time management are:

• improved quality of work and improved quality of care.

• having enough time to do special things for patients, such as styling hair, applying makeup, polishing nails, or accompanying a patient to the chapel or for a walk outside the facility.

• having the ability to get more done in less time.

• feeling as if you have an enjoyable and satisfying job, and feeling better about work you do.

• feeling positive about your contributions to the facility and to patient care.

• feeling less stressed than previously.

• having energy and not feeling exhausted at the end of the day.

Suggestions for Time Management

Remember that while you are at work, you are on duty. You are being paid to work the whole time. If you run out of things to do, help your coworkers or do things that need to be done on your unit. Do these things without being told. Develop a personal time management plan by using the

APIE system and trying the following suggestions:

- Make rounds on your assigned patients as soon as possible after report. During this round, identify patient needs and problems, and meet immediate needs that cannot wait, such as assisting a patient to the bathroom.
  —By the end of this round, you should have a mental plan for the care of each patient, and have a basic idea of things the patient needs during your shift. You do this by combining information learned in report and while receiving your assignment with what you learned during your rounds.
  —Write things down. Always have a pen and notepad with you to record important information and observations.
  —Remember patient needs and requests or write them down.
  —Take advantage of and use facility or unit organizational tools.

- If you have not already done so, after report, you should make sure you have clear instructions and care plan information needed to care for your patients.

- Develop a routine for things you do each day, such as reporting, making rounds, and collecting information, such as intake and output at the end of the shift.
  —Make a list of your assigned patients and identify their needs.
  —Plan for high-need patients who will require more time.
  —Identify patients with higher-level needs, including those who will need extra time because of illness, demanding behavior, need for terminal care, frequent monitoring, or other problems. Incorporate the extra time needed by

these patients into your plan. You will need to spend more time with these patients, and will make more trips to their rooms. However, you must find a way to do these things without ignoring the needs of the other patients in your assignment, so planning is very important.
  —Set goals for times by which certain tasks must be completed; watch the clock to see if you are meeting this goal. If not, modify the plan, pick up your pace, or ask for help.

- Plan and organize your work
  —Write down your plan; make a new "to do" list each day.

- Plan for jobs for which you will need extra help or equipment. Arrange and agree on a time when this is convenient for all parties.
  —Plan for and agree on times when you will need to be available to help other workers.

- Set priorities for your shift, even though they may change.
  —Keep your plan flexible and expect the unexpected.
  —Devise a strategy and method for assigning priorities by asking yourself questions, such as the what, where, when, why, who, and how of your priorities.
  —Identify events that must be done by specific times, versus things you can take care of later.
  —Control the timing of events and care. Estimate where you should be at given times in your shift. Check the clock and see if you are meeting your goals. If not, determine why. Challenge yourself to improve on your time, or modify your plan to make it more realistic.
  —Emergencies, new admissions, and patient or family demands

are imposed on you by others. On most days, these things will not burden you if you do a good job in managing your time for events you can control.

—Focus on the patients' needs instead of tasks needing to be done. Focusing on patient needs helps you to attend to the tasks with far less stress and more job satisfaction.

—Constantly evaluate your efficiency and time management skills and work to improve them.

• Set goals to ensure the most important priorities are done.

—Without deadlines your goals are just dreams; make sure your deadlines are realistic and achievable.

—Remember that patients' physical needs always come first. For example, stocking the linen cart can wait until you have taken Mrs. Huynh to the bathroom.

—Complete high- or top-priority jobs immediately.

—Begin the next level priorities immediately after you have finished with top priorities.

—Set goals for checkpoints, or where you should be with your work at various times, such as having all baths given by 11 AM, or another time that is reasonable, considering your assignment. These checkpoint times may vary from one day to the next, depending on the acuity and needs of your patients.

• Avoid repetition. Plan to do like jobs at the same time, and make sure to finish them. Do them right the first time to prevent the need to redo them.

• Before beginning a task, organize what you will need.

• If you expect to be tied up for a while, such as while giving a bedbath and making an occupied bed, try to determine whether your other patients will need your assistance. If so, tend to their needs first, and explain you will return as soon as you can.

• Anticipate your supply needs and patients' personal needs. Anticipating and meeting patient needs without being asked may save a great deal of time.

• Bring necessary items to the room before beginning care so you will not have to waste time and energy retrieving forgotten items. Use your energy efficiently; avoid backtracking.

• Save trips by taking things with you. For example, you are passing fresh drinking water when Mr. Dombrowski's call signal goes on. Bring fresh water with you when you answer his light.

• Set time limits for tasks you must complete, such as taking vital signs, passing towels and fresh drinking water, or collecting intake and output information at the end of your shift. Determine the approximate time you should finish and stay on track.

—Avoid becoming distracted. Focus on what you are doing.

—Break routine tasks and jobs down into smaller, more manageable pieces, if possible.

—Try to break your own record for completing time consuming tasks. However, do not sacrifice safety and quality of care for the sake of speed. In trying to beat your own best record, be sure that doing so is safe. The time you save is not worth the price you pay for making an error. If cutting corners is the only way to save time, try modifying your routine. If you can streamline routine tasks by a minute each day, you have saved time.

- Communicate with peers, colleagues, and subordinates throughout your shift. Good communication is essential to unit operations and quality care.
  —Be tactful and polite in all communications.
  —Treat others with respect and integrity.
- Take breaks at appropriate times; you need the rest and relaxation; avoid bringing work on your break. Make sure you return to the unit on time.
- Avoid wasting time; remain organized so you make good use of your time.
- Avoid wasting time by visiting and gossiping with coworkers when on duty.
- Check on your patients while you are out and about on the unit. Look in the doors to be sure the patients are not in need.
  —Always ask patients if they need anything else before leaving the room.
  —Note whether your assigned patients are sick, unstable, or displaying behavior problems; develop a plan for nursing assistant action or intervention. Inform the nurse.
  —If you are behind in your work and cannot find a way to get caught up, consult the nurse.
  —If things are not going well for a specific patient, ask others for their opinions on the situation. They work closely with the patients, and may hesitate to volunteer the information. However, they may respond if asked.

Your coworkers may have insight into the cause of the problem or know a potential solution. Soliciting their input shows you value them as team members, and enhances their self-esteem.

- Practice good communication skills with patients and families while making rounds; this will save you time and prevent them calling you to the room later. Let them know you are on top of their loved one's condition and needs.
  —Stop to visit for a few minutes when you can. Do not wait for patients or families to seek you out. You are busy, and this seems like a time waster, but in the long run, it promotes satisfaction, and may save you time. Offer simple information to family members. Do not wait for them to question you. For example, "Your mother ate a good breakfast today," "The night nurse said your father had a restful night," and "Your auntie really enjoy her visit from the church members yesterday."
  —Family caregivers usually know the patient better than the nursing staff. Do not be afraid to ask them questions.
  —Avoid becoming defensive if family members express concerns about patient conditions. Listen to what they have to say. Tell them what you will do about their concern, and give them a follow up time if needed, such as, "I will check back in 30 minutes to see if she needs to use the bathroom." Thank them for sharing their concern. Inform the nurse promptly.
- Determine which patients require assessment versus those who require monitoring.

—Assessment is systematic or focused; it involves a thorough examination and investigation of a problem or potential problem. If you believe a problem warrants assessment, notify the nurse.

—Monitoring is simple oversight, such as looking in on or speaking with a patient, taking or reviewing vital signs, and addressing known problems. These activities are all within the scope of the nursing assistants' responsibilities.

• You are a member of a team. You depend on your coworkers to help you. You must also be willing to help them when they need it.

• If you see something that needs to be done, do it without being told.

• All staff are responsible for answering call signals, even if the patient is not part of your assignment.

Good time management is a valuable skill to possess. Avoid losing your focus. Ensuring quality patient care is the greatest priority. By using the APIE process to enhance your time management skills, you can make a difference in your job satisfaction and patient care.

INFECTION

Infections are caused by micro-organisms and can be:

- Local (confined to one area)—such as a boil or skin abscess
- Generalized—such as pneumonia (in the lungs)
- Systemic—widespread through the bloodstream (bacteremia)

BACTERIAL INFECTIONS

Bacteria are simple one-celled microbes. They cause infections in the skin, respiratory tract, urinary tract, and bloodstream. An example is *Staphylococcus aureus*. Staphylococci cause many infections such as:

- Surgical wound infections
- Abscesses
- Boils
- Toxic shock

Bacteria are often the cause of serious skin, respiratory, urinary, and gastrointestinal infections in patients. If the physician suspects that a patient has a bacterial infection, a culture and sensitivity test may be ordered. This test can be done on urine, drainage from a wound, blood, or other body fluid. The culture tells the physician what type of microbe is causing the infection. The sensitivity tells the physician which antibiotic (antibacterial drug) should be used to treat the infection.

Tuberculosis

People at risk for tuberculosis infection include those who:

- Are HIV positive
- Are infected but fail to take their medication for the full treatment period
- Live in poverty and are malnourished
- Have immigrated to the United States from countries where tuberculosis is still common
- Have inactive tuberculosis and have grown older. The immune system weakens to the point where it can no longer contain the pathogen.

Infection occurs when the bacteria enter the body through the lungs. As the disease progresses, the person will show one or more of the following signs and symptoms:

- Fatigue
- Loss of appetite and weight
- Weakness
- Elevated temperature in the afternoon and evening
- Night sweats
- Spitting up blood (hemoptysis)
- Coughing

The infection can be spread through droplets in respiratory secretions.

Diagnosis

The presence of tuberculosis bacteria in the body can be shown by:

- A sputum culture—grows the organisms from a specimen of secretions from the person's lungs
- Chest x-rays—show the extent of the disease process in the lungs

- A positive skin test (Mantoux test)—shows the presence of antibodies to the tuberculosis organisms in the body

Treatment

A combination of drugs is often used to control the infection because many organisms have become resistant to specific drugs. Once drug therapy begins, the patient usually becomes noncontagious within 2 to 3 weeks. The therapy continues for 6 months to 2 years.

Escherichia coli 0157:H7

E.coli is transmitted:
- In contaminated and undercooked meat
- In produce that has been rinsed in water contaminated with cattle feces
- In produce handled by a person who has been handling contaminated food
- On contaminated cutting boards and utensils
- In unpasteurized milk and apple juice
- In pools and lakes contaminated with fecal matter

Signs and Symptoms

After 1 to 2 days:
- Watery diarrhea
- Nausea
- Vomiting
- Cramping

After another 1 or 2 days:
- The diarrhea becomes bloody.
- The abdomen becomes distended (enlarged) and very tender.
- Dehydration may become obvious.
- There may be petechiae, small purplish spots on the body surface, caused by minute hemorrhages.

The diarrhea may subside in 5 to 7 days, but the condition injures the mucous membranes, causing the pathogen to escape into the bloodstream. The patient develops signs and symptoms of serious illness, such as:
- Decreased urine output that may progress to complete renal failure
- Mental confusion
- Seizures (convulsions)
- Muscle weakness
- Pain and numbness of the feet and legs

This bacterial infection can be deadly. Treatment is supportive, and the patient requires careful monitoring. Water intake is very important, but liquid intake will require very close observation because of the potential for kidney damage.

OTHER SIGNIFICANT BACTERIA

Klebsiella is a bacterium that is a major cause of pneumonia, urinary tract, and wound infections. The bacteria are quickly becoming drug resistant. Klebsiella normally resides in the colon, where it is used for normal bowel function. If it escapes from the colon and enters an area where it does not belong, serious infection occurs. Klebsiella usually infects patients with weakened immune systems.

Listeriosis is caused by ingesting the *Listeria monocytogenes* bacteria in contaminated food. The bacterium is found in some raw foods, such as uncooked meats and vegetables, hot dogs, cold cuts, soft cheeses, and unpasteurized (raw) milk. It is killed by pasteurization and cooking, but in some foods such as hot dogs, contamination may occur after cooking but before packaging.

Acinetobacter baumannii is a bacterium that experienced a revival due to the war in Iraq. It has not been commonly seen since the Vietnam war. Carriers have been returning from Iraq with this pathogen on their skin, although they show no signs of infection. It is a common cause of pneumonia. Pneumonia caused by this organism has a high mortality rate. It also causes infections of the bone, bloodstream, and internal organs, which complicate patient care. There are few drugs to treat it, and no new medicines are in development.

Streptococcus A is a bacterium that produces very powerful enzymes that destroy tissue and blood cells. Most carriers have no symptoms. They pass the infection to others by coughing or sneezing, or by touching a susceptible person or environmental surface without washing their hands. Strep A causes a serious skin infection called necrotizing fasciitis. This condition is also called "flesh-eating" or "man-eating" strep. The pathogen can enter a break as tiny as a paper cut. Once inside the body, the patient develops flu-like illness. Pain in the area of the broken skin is often severe, and out of proportion to the injury.

The injury worsens rapidly over several days. The toxin destroys muscle tissue. Pain increases, and severe swelling and redness develop on the skin. At this point, it can spread as much as an inch an hour, causing tissue death. Blood cannot reach or nourish the dead tissue. The wound turns black and gangrenous, requiring amputation. Strep A can be so serious that although the patient survives, he or she is scarred and has as many as all four extremities amputated. Every system of the body can fail as a result of the severe infection and toxicity of the pathogen. It causes massive shock, heart and respiratory failure, low blood pressure, and renal failure. Good handwashing helps reduce the risk of infection. Prompt diagnosis and treatment of this condition are essential because the infection spreads rapidly. About 25 percent of cases result in death.

SPORES

Spores are microscopic reproductive bodies that are responsible for the spread of some diseases. They can survive in a dormant form until conditions are ideal for reproduction. The spores will multiply and continue to spread infection. They are very difficult to eliminate.

Norovirus (Norwalk virus) is a highly contagious pathogen that causes infectious diarrhea. You may have heard of these viruses on the news. Many cruise ships had diarrhea outbreaks caused by *Norovirus*. Very few virus particles are needed to transmit infection. The pathogen originates in the stool. The viruses are highly resistant to disinfectants used for cleaning environmental surfaces. They are also highly resistant to alcohol-based handwashing agents. *Norovirus* remains active on the hands for at least four hours, on hard dry surfaces for ten days, and on wet surfaces for weeks.

Patients with infectious diarrhea will be placed on contact precautions. When caring for patients with infectious diarrhea, and other conditions known or suspected to be spread by spores, such as *C. Difficile, Norovirus, Anthrax,* and *Botulism,* you must use good handwashing. The friction and running water will remove spores and viruses from your hands. *Do not use alcohol hand cleaners, which will not eliminate the spores on your hands or in the environment.*

Aspergillosis is a serious fungal infection that is also spread by spores. It affects patients with weakened immune systems, such as those with HIV and AIDS, cancer patients, and transplant patients. An infection in the bloodstream can be deadly, and few drugs are available to treat it. There are more than 150 species of *Aspergillus* genus, but only a few are harmful. Most healthy people are immune to this fungus.

VIRAL INFECTIONS

A virus is the smallest microbe and has a variety of shapes. Common viral infections include hepatitis, herpes, AIDS, chickenpox, influenza, common cold, measles, and mumps.

Herpes zoster

Shingles (herpes zoster) occurs in people who were infected by the virus that causes chickenpox. The organisms did not leave the body. They remained hidden in the nervous system in a nonactive state. Years later, when the person is in a weakened condition, the organisms become active. Painful blisterlike lesions develop in the skin along the paths of sensitive nerves. The blisters contain infectious organisms. Workers who have never had chickenpox, and those who have not been immunized against chickenpox should not care for a person with shingles.

Influenza

Influenza (or flu) is caused by a family of viruses. The infection can lead to serious consequences for elderly or frail people. Vaccines offer some protection against influenza viruses and are given to residents in long-term care.

Someone with the flu may experience:
- Malaise (general unwell feeling)
- Chills
- Fever
- Muscle aches and pains
- Coldlike symptoms

The virus may also lower the patient's resistance to other infectious organisms. These can cause pneumonia and other life-threatening infections. Antibiotics may be given to combat bacterial infections that may develop.

You can help patients in your care by:
- Staying healthy
- Not reporting for duty when you are ill
- Carrying out standard precautions faithfully
- Following the facility's policies regarding special precautions when a patient has a respiratory infection
- Encouraging the patient to drink fluids
- Reporting to the nurse when a visitor seems to be ill

Hepatitis

Hepatitis is an inflammation of the liver caused by several viruses, including:
- Hepatitis A virus
- Hepatitis B virus
- Hepatitis C virus
- Hepatitis D virus
- Hepatitis E virus
- Hepatitis G virus

The various types of hepatitis are summarized in Table 5-1.

Table 5-1 TYPES OF HEPATITIS INFECTIONS

TYPE	MODE OF TRANSMISSION	SIGNS & SYMPTOMS	VACCINE	U.S. STATISTICS	TREATMENT	COMMENTS
hepatitis A	Oral/fecal; on hands or transferred to food	Abdominal pain, loss of appetite, fatigue, nausea, diarrhea, dark urine, jaundice	Vaccine available; immune globulin used for short-term immunity	125,000 to 200,000 cases and approx. 100 deaths annually	Bedrest and limited activity for up to 30 days	Usually lasts less than 2 months; not a chronic condition
hepatitis B	Blood and body fluid; mother to fetus	Abdominal pain, loss of appetite, fatigue, nausea, diarrhea, dark urine, jaundice	Vaccine available	140,000 to 320,000 total infections; approx. 5,000 to 6,000 deaths annually	Most recover within 6 months; For chronic cases, Interferon	Over 1 million chronically infected; Can lead to cirrhosis or liver cancer
hepatitis C	Blood and body fluid; mother to fetus	Mostly asymptomatic; patient may have abdominal pain, loss of appetite, fatigue, nausea, diarrhea, dark urine, jaundice	None	28,000 to 180,000 total infections; approx. 10,000 deaths annually	Interferon; effective in approx. 33% of patients	Approx. 4 million chronically infected; can lead to cirrhosis or liver cancer. Varies between first and second place on the annual list of leading causes of liver transplant in U.S. Most carriers are asymptomatic for many years before learning of infection.
hepatitis D	Blood and body fluid	Abdominal pain, loss of appetite, fatigue, nausea, diarrhea, dark urine, jaundice	Hepatitis B vaccine	Approx. 5,000 infections annually	Interferon may be effective in some patients	Develops only in the presence of hepatitis B or acquired simultaneously with HBV; few chronic cases. 70% to 80% develop cirrhosis.

hepatitis E	Oral/fecal; contaminated water	Abdominal pain, loss of appetite, fatigue, nausea, diarrhea, dark urine, jaundice	None	Rare in U.S.	Rest, limited activity for 2 weeks	Almost all U.S. cases are in travelers returning from high risk areas, primarily Mexico, Asia, Africa. Few chronic cases.
hepatitis G Also known as GB virus-C (GBV-C)	Blood Also believed to be sexually transmitted, IV drug use, tattoo needles, maternal to fetus	Most patients are asymptomatic	None	900 to 2,000 cases annually	Rest	First identified in 1996, and more research is necessary. Some experts believe that this virus is not responsible for clinically significant cases of hepatitis. Others note that the virus can be identified by a blood test, but does not cause illness. Dialysis patients are at high risk. Believed to be persistent in 15–30% of cases.

Acquired Immune Deficiency Syndrome (AIDS)

AIDS is a viral disease. It is transmitted primarily through direct contact with the bodily secretions of an infected person. The virus that causes AIDS is the human immunodeficiency virus (HIV). The ways in which HIV is transmitted include:
- Blood to blood through:
  - Transfusion of infected blood. Note that federal regulations prevent the use of untested and unregulated blood in the United States.
  - Treatment of hemophilia with clotting factor from infected blood.
  - Needle sharing among drug users.
  - Prick from a contaminated needle or sharp.
  - Unsterile instruments used for procedures such as ear piercing or tattooing.
- Unprotected vaginal, oral, or anal intercourse when one partner is infected
- Infected mother to infant during:
  - Pregnancy
  - Birth process
  - Nursing (breastfeeding)

The AIDS virus (HIV):
- Has many variants
- Does not live for long outside of the body
- Is affected by common chemicals such as bleach
- Depresses the body's immune system
- Makes the infected person more susceptible to infections
- Makes the infected person more likely to experience complications such as:
  - *Pneumocystis carinii* pneumonia—a serious lung infection
  - Kaposi's sarcoma—a serious malignancy affecting many body organs
  - Brain involvement leading to dementia
  - Eye involvement leading to blindness
  - Tuberculosis
  - Other opportunistic infections

Symptoms of HIV Infection

When they do appear, symptoms consist of:
- Acute flulike symptoms
- Fever
- Night sweats
- Fatigue
- Swollen lymph nodes
- Sore throat
- Gastrointestinal problems
- Headache

Treatment

No specific treatment is able to cure AIDS at the present time. A combination of drugs currently in use reduces both the symptoms and viral activity.
- No vaccine prevents the infection from developing.
- Nutritional and other forms of preventive therapy are aimed at maintaining a person with AIDS in the best health possible.
- Therapy is directed toward vigorously treating each infection as it appears.
- The drugs do not cure the disease. They slow its progression. When patients fail to take their drug protocol exactly, the disease state returns quickly and more strongly than before.
- There is no evidence that AIDS is transmitted:
  - Through kissing, touching, or hugging an HIV-infected person

- By eating at the same table with an infected person
- By using the same toilet seat
- Through insect bites

Hantavirus

- Spread by contact with rodents (rats and mice) or their excretions, including urine and stool
- Once disturbed, viral particles in the excretions become airborne and can be inhaled

Signs and Symptoms

These appear 1 to 5 weeks later and can include:

- High fever
- Chills
- Muscle aches
- Cough
- Nausea
- Vomiting
- Diarrhea
- Dizziness
- Lethargy

- As the disease progresses, the patient becomes very short of breath and seriously ill. Respiratory support may be necessary.
- The virus is not spread person to person.
- Spread of *Hantavirus* can be reduced by preventing rodents from entering the home or eliminating them if they are present.

Severe Acute Respiratory Syndrome

Severe acute respiratory syndrome (SARS) is a viral respiratory illness caused by a coronavirus that appeared in China in late 2002. It has spread around the world and is highly contagious. Much remains to be learned about this condition. SARS seems to spread by very close person-to-person contact by inhaling and touching respiratory droplets. It may also be spread by the airborne method; this is being researched. SARS is treated similarly to serious pneumonia. Antiviral drugs are given and respirations are supported. Your facility will require frequent handwashing and special isolation precautions.

FUNGAL INFECTIONS

Two groups of fungi are most commonly associated with infection in humans:

- Yeasts. These can affect areas of the body such as the mouth (*Candida albicans*), vagina (*Candida albicans*), and skin (*Tinea capitis*).
- Molds. A common mold that can cause infection in the lungs of humans is called *Aspergillus.*

Coccidioidomycosis (Valley Fever)

This illness is caused by *Coccidioides immitis*. It occurs primarily as a respiratory infection and is seldom fatal in otherwise healthy people. In people with immunosuppression, however, the death rate is high. The illness is treated with antibiotics.

PROTOZOAL INFECTIONS

Protozoa are simple one-celled organisms that live on living matter. They cause diseases such as:

- Malaria
- Toxoplasmosis
- African sleeping sickness
- Amebiasis

Giardiasis

Giardiasis is caused by *Giardia lamblia,* which is found in the water supplies of many communities. It causes severe diarrhea. This pathogen is also spread by spores.

Cryptosporidiosis

Cryptosporidiosis is caused by *Cryptosporidium* protozoa, which are found in the digestive tracts of domestic animals and are transferred by contact. It causes severe diarrhea, especially in immunosuppressed people. Avoid alcohol hand cleanser if this organism is present; use soap and water for handwashing.

Signs and Symptoms

Some signs and symptoms of diseases caused by protozoa include:
- Diarrhea
- Dysentery (infection in the lower bowel)
- Encephalitis (inflammation of the brain)

PARASITES

You have learned that yeast and mold are opportunistic parasites. *Parasites* survive and thrive by feeding off a human or animal. Fleas and ticks are common examples of parasites.

Head Lice

Head lice are parasites that spread primarily by direct contact with an infected person. They can also be spread by sharing personal belongings such as brushes, combs, ribbons, caps, clothing, and bedding with others. You cannot contract head lice from pets and animals. The lice do not hop, jump, or fly, but they can crawl very quickly. When performing hair care, check patients for *nits,* which are tiny, oval shaped eggs that are yellow-white in color. They look like dandruff, but are firmly attached to the hair and are very difficult to remove. Dandruff

brushes off readily, whereas nits do not. The nits will hatch into live lice. Lice are tiny brown insects about the size of a sesame seed. They run away from light quickly. Notify the nurse for further assessment if you notice nits or other abnormalities.

If nits or lice are suspected, you must wear a gown and gloves for contact with the patient until the patient has been treated. You must also wear gloves and a gown when handling the patient's clothing or linen. The physician will order a medicated shampoo to kill the parasites. Contact precautions will be used for 24 hours after the patient is treated. It is important to remove all of the nits, as the shampoo may not kill them. A special comb is used for this time-consuming task. To be effective, all the nits must be removed from the scalp, or the nits will hatch, producing more lice. You may be directed to check other patients for the presence of head lice.

Scabies

Scabies is a disease of the skin caused by a parasite called a *mite.* A mite is a microscopic organism that cannot be seen with the eye. Scabies is highly contagious and is spread by direct and indirect contact. It causes a rash and severe itching of the skin. The rash is usually in the:
- webs of the fingers.
- inside the wrists.
- outside the elbows.
- underarm, waist, and nipple areas.
- genital area in men.
- knees and lower buttocks.

The patient will be placed in contact precautions. You may be directed to apply a medicated lotion to the patient's entire body, not just the rash area. Avoid the patient's eyelids or lips and wear a gown and gloves when applying this treatment. The lotion remains on the patient's skin for 12 to 24 hours, then is washed off in the tub or shower. If the patient's hands are washed during this period, reapply the lotion. Depending on the solution used, another treatment may be required several days to several weeks later. It takes about a month from the first treatment for the rash to disappear. The patient may experience itching even after the scabies are eliminated. You may be directed to check other patients for the appearance of a rash. Facility personnel may also be treated to prevent the spread of the mite.

Bedbugs (Cimex Lectularius)

Bedbugs are parasites that have been found throughout the world, with the exception of Antarctica. They are usually seen at night, are stealthy and fast-moving, and multiply quickly. They can survive in hot and cold environments. Although there is no recorded incidence of disease as a result of bedbugs, they are parasites that bite, causing a painful, rash type area on the skin. The bedbugs use their mouth parts, which have adapted to piercing skin to obtain its blood meal. Bedbugs have an anticoagulant in their saliva that prevents blood from clotting when they are eating. Some people are very sensitive to this substance, and have an allergic skin reaction. Others can live with bed bugs and not be aware of them. Some people develop welts that look like flea or mosquito bites. They look like tiny, red bumps, and they itch. The bites may appear in lines, similar to scabies. Adult bedbugs can survive for up to a year without eating. Like lice and scabies, some bedbugs are resistant to over-the-counter insecticides, and setting off pesticide bombs may scatter rather than kill them.

A bedbug is tiny, a little smaller than a pencil eraser. They are flat, and clear or white in appearance before feeding. After eating a blood meal, they develop a red-brown hue. They leave little excretion droppings on the sheets and may give off a sickly sweet smell. Finding tiny bloodstains on the linen from crushed bugs, or dark spots from the droppings is a strong indication that bedbugs are present. They hide in the seams of clothing and furnishings, so the patient may have brought them from home and not be aware of it. They may hide in cracks and crevices in mattresses, bed frames, behind headboards, inside nightstands, behind baseboards, window and door casings, pictures, and moldings. They have also been found hiding in furniture and clutter, such as piles of books, papers, boxes, and items near sleeping areas. Shining a flashlight and aiming a hot hair dryer into crevices forces the insects out.

If bedbugs are noted, a professional exterminator must be called to eliminate them. Everything in the room must be cleaned and washed. Items that cannot be washed should be sealed in plastic bags and exposed to very hot or freezing temperatures. The bugs' eggs also must be found and eliminated, or more bugs will hatch. If you suspect bedbugs in a patient's room, inform the nurse immediately.

INFECTION CONTROL

SPREAD OF INFECTION

The development of infection is dangerous for patients and very costly to the insurance carrier and the hospital. Prevention of infection is a major nursing assistant function.

Transmission is a term used to describe how microbes travel about. In the study of infection control, we are concerned with the transmission of *pathogens,* the harmful microbes that can cause disease. Pathogens are transmitted in hospitals by several routes, and one pathogen may have multiple methods of travel, or modes of spreading. To prevent infection, workers must anticipate the spread and block all the potential methods of transmission. This is done by using good handwashing technique and applying the infection control techniques and precautions in this chapter. Infection is transmitted (spread) by several methods. These are the:

- *airborne method*—Pathogens spread by the airborne method are very tiny and light in weight. They enter the air in respiratory secretions, or mucus from the nose, mouth, and lungs containing the pathogens. A cough or sneeze expels the pathogens into the air. Because they are so lightweight, they can travel long distances through the ventilation system, in dust, or on moisture particles in the air. Because of their weight, these pathogens do not drop to the ground quickly and are easily inhaled by others.

- *droplet method*—*Droplets* also are respiratory secretions, such as those produced by sneezing, coughing, or blowing the nose. The pathogens spread by droplets are larger and heavier than those spread by the airborne method. Because of their size and weight, they usually do not spread beyond three feet from the carrier. Thus, if you are standing on the opposite side of the room, you are less likely to inhale a pathogen if a patient sneezes than you would be if you were giving him or her a bath. Understanding the difference between the airborne and droplet methods of transmission is important so you can follow proper procedures to prevent infection from spreading.

- *common vehicle method*—Common vehicles are an additional means of transferring pathogens from one person to another. If a pathogen enters a common vehicle, such as food, water, or medications, many people are likely to be infected when they eat or drink the substance.

- *vector method*—Vectors are insects and small animals that can carry pathogens. A wide variety of insects and parasites are vectors. Common examples are flies, roaches, mosquitos, ticks, and fleas. However, parasites such as scabies and body lice also are vectors, as are small and larger animals, such as reptiles, mice, rats, bats, cats, and dogs. Vectors can transmit infection by biting or licking the skin of the susceptible host, or by carrying the pathogens on an area of their bodies where you pick them up on your hands through direct or indirect contact.

- *direct contact method*—When this method is used, the transfer of pathogens occurs by touching an infected person, such as when shaking hands. You pick up the pathogen on your hand, then introduce it to your body.

- *indirect contact method*—The indirect contact method involves touching environmental surfaces and objects, such as doorknobs, faucet handles, soiled linen, or other items on which the invisible pathogens are present. As with direct contact, you pick up the pathogen on your hands, then later introduce it to your body.

- *fomite method*—Fomites are any supply items or equipment that are implicated in indirect contact transmission. Examples of fomites are linen, bedpans, urinals, and other supplies with invisible pathogens on them. You pick up the pathogen on your hands and spread it to the inside of your body through nonintact skin or by touching your mucous membranes.

CHAIN OF INFECTION

Understanding the chain of infection is important because the methods used to break the chain protect you, the patients, visitors, and other workers. In fact, infection control information is among the most important information you will study in your nursing assistant program. If any part of the chain of infection is broken, the disease will not spread.

Figure 6-1 shows examples of how the various links in the chain can be broken. The purpose of medical asepsis, infection control, standard precautions, and other procedures or techniques is to break the links in the chain. This will immediately interrupt the essential factors and prevent the infection from spreading.

Links in the Chain

A *carrier* is a person who is infected with a pathogen, infection, or disease that can be spread to others. He or she may or may not know of the infection. This is why we use various methods of precautions for all patients without regard for disease or diagnosis. A person may look normal and healthy, when in fact he or she is a carrier of a significant pathogen. The *chain of infection* describes six factors necessary for an infection to develop. Each link in the chain represents one factor that is essential to the spread of infection. All six factors must be present for the infection to spread. The links represent the:

- *causative agent*—the pathogen that can cause infection or disease in humans.
- *source* or *reservoir*—the place where the pathogen can live, multiply, and survive.
  —The *source* can be a person, animal, or substance from which the infectious agent passes to the susceptible host. It may also be an inanimate object, such as water, a sink or countertop, or doorknob.
  —The *reservoir may be the same as the source or different from the source.* This is because the reservoir is where the pathogen lives or resides, while the source is the site from which the pathogen is transferred to others. (This distinction is important

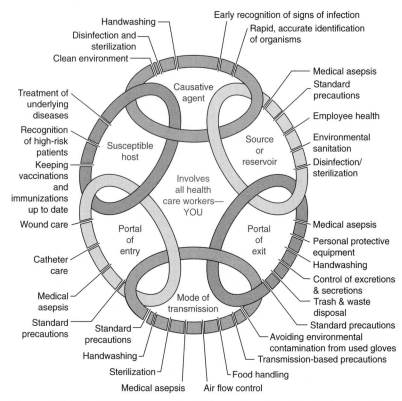

Figure 6-1 The circles represent the links to the chain of infection. Breaking a link by using any of the methods listed will prevent the infection from spreading.

when deciding the types of precautions and control measures to use to prevent further spread of infection.)

- *susceptible host*—the person who can become infected because he or she lacks immunity or physical resistance to overcome the invasion of pathogens.
- *mode (method) of transmission*—the method by which the disease is spread. Some diseases can be spread by more than one method.
- *portal of entry*—the location where the microbe enters the body, such as a tiny cut or crack in the skin, or

mucous membranes of the eyes, nose, mouth, or genital area.

- *portal of exit*—blood or body fluids, secretions, excretions, or droplets in which the pathogens travel when they leave the body.

STANDARD PRECAUTIONS

Standard precautions are used for all patient care (Figure 6-2). When patients are known to have or are suspected of having an infectious disease, transmission-based precautions (Table 6-1) are used in addition to standard precautions.

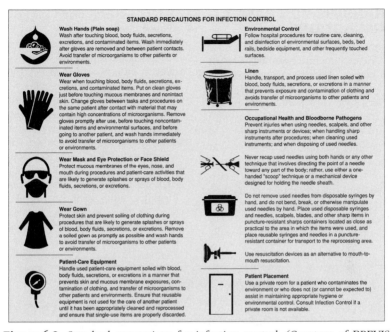

Figure 6-2   Standard precautions for infection control. (Courtesy of BREVIS Corporation, Salt Lake City, UT.)

Table 6-1   TRANSMISSION-BASED PRECAUTIONS FOR COMMON DISEASES

TRANSMISSION-BASED PRECAUTIONS CATEGORY	DISEASE OR CONDITION
Airborne	Tuberculosis Measles
Airborne and contact	Chickenpox Widespread shingles
Droplet	German measles Mumps Influenza
Contact	Head or body lice, scabies Impetigo Infected pressure ulcer with heavy drainage

TRANSMISSION-BASED PRECAUTIONS

- Airborne precautions—used for diseases that are transmitted by air currents. The pathogens are small and light and are suspended in the air or on dust particles in the air. They can travel a long distance from the source (Figure 6-3).

- Droplet precautions—used for diseases that can be spread by means of large droplets in the air. A person can spread droplets containing infectious pathogens by sneezing, coughing, talking, singing, or laughing. The droplets generally do not travel more than 3 feet from the source (Figure 6-4).

- Contact precautions—used when the infectious pathogen is spread by direct or indirect contact. Direct contact occurs when the caregiver touches a contaminated area on the patient's skin or blood or body fluids containing the infectious pathogen. Indirect contact occurs when the caregiver touches items contaminated with the infectious material, such as the patient's personal belongings, equipment or supplies used in the care of the patient, contaminated linens, and so on (Figure 6-5).

AIRBORNE PRECAUTIONS
(in addition to Standard Precautions)

VISITORS: Report to nurse before entering.

Patient Placement
Use **private room** that has:
Monitored negative air pressure,
6 to 12 air changes per hour,
Discharge of air outdoors or HEPA filtration if recirculated.
Keep room door closed and patient in room.

Respiratory Protection
Wear an N95 respirator when entering the room of a patient with known or suspected infectious pulmonary **tuberculosis.**
Susceptible persons should not enter the room of patients known or suspected to have **measles** (rubeola) or **varicella** (chickenpox) if other immune caregivers are available. If susceptible persons must enter, they should wear an **N95 respirator.** (Respirator or surgical mask not required if immune to measles and varicella.)

Patient Transport
Limit transport of patient from room to essential purposes only. Use **surgical mask** on patient during transport.

Figure 6-3 Airborne precautions. (Courtesy of BREVIS Corporation, Salt Lake City, UT.)

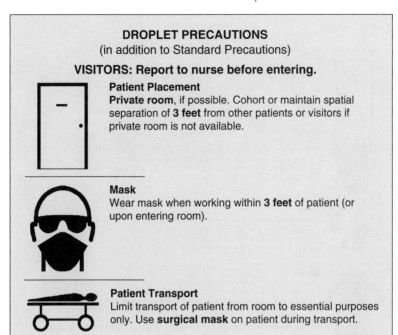

DROPLET PRECAUTIONS
(in addition to Standard Precautions)

VISITORS: Report to nurse before entering.

Patient Placement
Private room, if possible. Cohort or maintain spatial separation of **3 feet** from other patients or visitors if private room is not available.

Mask
Wear mask when working within **3 feet** of patient (or upon entering room).

Patient Transport
Limit transport of patient from room to essential purposes only. Use **surgical mask** on patient during transport.

Figure 6-4 Droplet precautions. (Courtesy of BREVIS Corporation, Salt Lake City, UT.)

PERSONAL PROTECTIVE EQUIPMENT (PPE)

Sequence for Applying PPE

1. Wash hands
2. Gown
3. Mask
4. Goggles or face shield
5. Gloves

Sequence for Removing PPE

1. Gloves
2. Wash hands
3. Goggles or face shield
4. Gown
5. Mask
6. Wash hands

See Table 6-2 for guidelines for using PPEs and Table 6-3 for the rules of infection control.

CONTACT PRECAUTIONS
(in addition to Standard Precautions)

VISITORS: Report to nurse before entering.

Patient Placement
Private room, if possible. Cohort if private room is not available.

Gloves
Wear gloves when entering patient room.
Change gloves after having contact with infective material that may contain high concentrations of microorganisms (**fecal** material and **wound drainage**). **Remove** gloves before leaving patient room.

Wash
Wash hands with an **antimicrobial** agent immediately after glove removal. After glove removal and handwashing, ensure that hands do not touch potentially contaminated environmental surfaces or items in the patient's room to avoid transfer of microorganisms to other patients or environments.

Gown
Wear gown when **entering** patient room if you anticipate that your clothing will have substantial contact with the patient, environmental surfaces, or items in the patient's room, or if the patient is **incontinent**, has **diarrhea**, an **ileostomy**, a **colostomy**, or **wound drainage** not contained by a dressing. **Remove** gown before leaving the patient's environment and ensure that clothing does not contact potentially contaminated environmental surfaces to avoid transfer of microorganisms to other patients or environments.

Patient Transport
Limit transport of patient to essential purposes only. During transport, ensure that precautions are maintained to minimize the risk of transmission of microorganisms to other patients and contamination of environmental surfaces and equipment.

Patient-Care Equipment
Dedicate the use of noncritical patient-care equipment to a single patient. If common equipment is used, clean and disinfect between patients.

Figure 6-5   Contact precautions. (Courtesy of BREVIS Corporation, Salt Lake City, UT.)

Table 6-2   PERSONAL PROTECTIVE EQUIPMENT IN COMMON NURSING ASSISTANT TASKS

Note: Use this chart as a general guideline only. Add protective equipment if special circumstances exist. Know and follow your facility policies for using personal protective equipment.

NURSING ASSISTANT TASK	GLOVES	GOWN	GOGGLES/ FACE SHIELD	SURGICAL MASK
Washing/rinsing utensils in the soiled utility room	Yes	Yes if splashing is likely	Yes if splashing is likely	Yes if splashing is likely
Holding pressure on a bleeding wound	Yes	Yes	Yes	Yes

Table 6-2   PERSONAL PROTECTIVE EQUIPMENT IN COMMON NURSING ASSISTANT TASKS (CONTINUED)

NURSING ASSISTANT TASK	GLOVES	GOWN	GOGGLES/ FACE SHIELD	SURGICAL MASK
Wiping the shower chair with disinfectant	Yes	No	No	No
Emptying a catheter bag	Yes	Yes if facility policy	Yes if facility policy	Yes if facility policy
Passing meal trays	No	No	No	No
Passing ice	No	No	No	No
Giving a backrub to a patient with a rash	Yes	No	No	No
Giving special mouth care to an unconscious patient	Yes	Yes if facility policy	Yes if facility policy	Yes if facility policy
Assisting with a dental procedure	Yes	Yes	Yes	Yes
Changing the bed after an incontinent patient has an episode of diarrhea	Yes	Yes	No	No
Taking an oral temperature with a glass thermometer (gloves are not necessary with an electronic thermometer unless this is your facility policy)	Yes	No	No	No
Taking a rectal temperature	Yes	No	No	No
Taking an axillary temperature	No	No	No	No
Taking a blood pressure	No	No	No	No
Assisting an alert patient to brush teeth	Yes	Yes if facility policy	Yes if facility policy	Yes if facility policy
Washing a patient's eyes	Yes	No	No	No
Giving perineal care	Yes	No	No	No
Washing the patient's abdomen when the skin is not broken	No	No	No	No
Washing the patient's arms when skin tears are present	Yes	No	No	No
Brushing a patient's dentures	Yes	No	No	No
Assisting the nurse while he or she suctions an unconscious patient with a tracheostomy	Yes	Yes	Yes	Yes

(continues)

Table 6-2   PERSONAL PROTECTIVE EQUIPMENT IN COMMON NURSING ASSISTANT TASKS (CONTINUED)

NURSING ASSISTANT TASK	GLOVES	GOWN	GOGGLES/ FACE SHIELD	SURGICAL MASK
Turning an incontinent patient who weighs 85 pounds	Yes if linen is soiled	Yes if your uniform will have substantial contact with the linen	No	No
Shaving a patient with a disposable razor	Yes, because this is a high-risk procedure	No	No	No
Shaving a patient with an electric razor	No	No	No	No
Cleaning the soiled utility room at the end of your shift	Yes	No	No	No

Table 6-3   RULES OF INFECTION CONTROL

DO

- Observe standard precautions and use barrier equipment (PPE) any time contact with blood, body fluids, secretions, excretions, mucous membranes, or nonintact skin is likely. Contact may be with a patient or an environmental surface.
- Clean up dishes immediately after use.
- Damp dust daily and be conscientious about cleaning while you carry out a task.
- Provide a bag for the disposal of used tissues.
- Turn the face to one side so that the assistant and the patient are not breathing directly on each other.
- Cover your nose and mouth when coughing or sneezing.
- Protect the skin on your hands by using warm water, drying thoroughly, and applying lotion if needed.
- Treat breaks in the skin immediately by washing thoroughly, cleaning with an antiseptic, and covering. Report any breaks in the skin to the nurse.
- Disinfect equipment that is used by more than one staff member or patient, such as a stethoscope, before and after each use.
- Gather or fold linen inward, with the dirtiest area toward the center.

TABLE 6-3   RULES OF INFECTION CONTROL (CONTINUED)

DO

- Clean reusable equipment immediately after use.
- Handle and dispose of soiled material according to facility policy.
- Practice good personal hygiene.
- Wash your hands frequently.
- Keep clean and dirty items separate in patient rooms and storage areas.
- Bring only needed items into the patient's room.
- Keep soiled linen and trash covered in closed containers.
- Perform procedures in the manner in which you were taught.
- Empty wastebaskets frequently, if this is your responsibility.

DO NOT

- Shake bed linens, because any microbes present could be released into the air.
- Allow dirty linen to touch your uniform.
- Eat or share food from a patient's tray.
- Borrow personal care items from another patient or employee.
- Permit the contents of bedpans or urinals to splash when being emptied.
- Report for duty if you have an infectious disease.
- Permit linen to touch the floor, which is always considered dirty.
- Carry clean linen against your uniform or bring more linen than necessary into the patient's room.
- Store lab specimens in the refrigerator with food.

CHAPTER

WHEN SOMETHING GOES WRONG

7

Disease (illness) is any change from a healthy state. Each illness has:

- An etiology—cause of the illness or abnormality
- A set of signs and symptoms, indicating that the illness is in progress
- A usual course or disease progression
- A prognosis or probable outcome of the illness

DISEASE TERMINOLOGY

- **Signs** of a disease can be seen by others.
- **Symptoms** are felt by the patient, who tells us about them.
- **Acute disease** develops suddenly, progresses rapidly, lasts for a predictable period, and then the person recovers or dies.
- **Chronic disease** often has periods when the patient experiences the signs and symptoms and periods when evidence of the disease is less pronounced or disappears altogether.
- **Ischemia** is the lack of adequate blood supply to a body tissue, which prevents delivery of essential oxygen and nutrients.
- **Congenital abnormalities** are abnormalities that are present at birth.

- **An acute exacerbation** of a chronic disease is when an increase in the severity of signs and symptoms occurs.
- **Inflammation** is a localized protective response of tissue to irritation, injury, or infection. It is characterized by redness, heat, swelling, pain, and sometimes loss of function.
- **Infection** is the invasion and proliferation of pathogens.
- **Autoimmune reaction** occurs when mechanisms that are for protection of the body turn against it and cause damage (e.g., rheumatoid arthritis, multiple sclerosis).
- **Irritations** abnormal sensitivity to stimulation, such as seeds in the intestinal tract or stones in the gallbladder or kidney.
- **Hypersensitivity reaction** is an allergic type of reaction such as hay fever, skin rashes, and asthma.
- **Metabolic imbalances** are conditions of fluid and electrolyte imbalance and include malnutrition, edema, scurvy, alcoholism, and diabetes mellitus.
- **Trauma** is an injury that causes tissue damage.
- **Neoplasm** is another term for tumor. A neoplasm is either benign or malignant (cancerous). Sometimes benign tumors can change and become malignant.

DISORDERS OF THE INTEGUMENTARY SYSTEM

8

DISORDERS

Skin Lesions

Injury or disease can cause changes in skin structures. These changes are called lesions. The lesions may be caused by disease, trauma, wear, or the aging process. When caring for patients with skin lesions, standard precautions are followed. Some of the most common skin lesions or eruptions are:

- Macules—flat, discolored spots, as in measles
- Nodules—small, knotlike protrusions, a small mass of tissue
- Papules—small, solid, raised spots, as in chickenpox
- Pustules—raised spots filled with pus, as in acne
- Vesicles—raised spots filled with watery fluid, such as a blister
- Wheals (or welts)—large, raised, irregular areas frequently associated with itching, as in hives
- Excoriations—portions of the skin that appear scraped or scratched away
- Crusts—areas of dried body secretions, such as scabs

Care of Skin Lesions

When skin lesions are present, take the following precautions when caring for patients.

- Closely observe the patient's skin on admission, but do not remove any dressings. Any changes noted

should be reported immediately and described accurately.
- Soap and water and rubbing lotions are often contraindicated (not permitted). Check the nursing care plan before bathing the patient or giving a backrub.
- Special products may be used for bathing or soaking the skin, such as colloidal oatmeal.
- Wear gloves when contact with blood, body fluids (including drainage from blisters or skin lesions), or nonintact skin is likely.
- Do not remove any crusts from skin lesions without permission from the nurse.
- Handle the patient gently. Avoid rubbing the skin.
- Special bed linen may be used, such as sterile linen, linen that has been washed in special detergent, or disposable linen. Special bedding will be listed on the care plan.
- A bed cradle may be placed on the bed to prevent the sheet from contacting the open skin areas.
- Notify the nurse if the:
  - Skin lesions are draining;
  - Drainage changes in color; or
  - Drainage increases; or
  - Drainage has a bad or foul odor.

Pressure Ulcers (Dermal Ulcers)

Pressure ulcers, commonly called bedsores or dermal ulcers, may occur in patients of any age. Pressure ulcers are caused by prolonged pressure on an area of the body that interferes with circulation. The tissue first becomes reddened. As the cells die (undergo necrosis) from lack of nourishment, the skin breaks down, and an ulcer forms. The resulting pressure ulcers may become large and deep.

Pressure ulcers occur most frequently over areas where bones come close to the surface (Figures 8-1, 8-2). Patients also tend to develop pressure ulcers where body parts rub and cause friction, for example, between the folds of the buttocks. The rubbing of tubing and other equipment used in the care of patients over a long period can also cause pressure ulcers.

Development of Pressure Ulcers

Tissue breakdown occurs in four stages. Nursing interventions at each

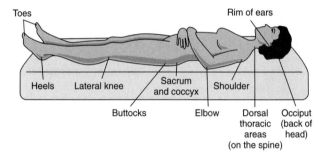

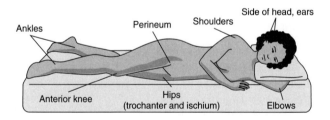

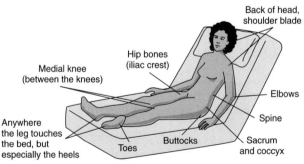

Figure 8-1 Common areas for pressure ulcers.

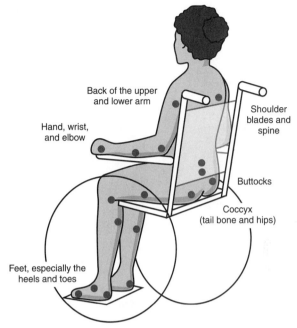

Figure 8-2   Common areas for pressure ulcers when sitting in a chair or wheelchair.

stage can limit the process and prevent further damage. Remember to continue all preventive measures throughout care.

Stage I (Figure 8-3A, B):

- The skin develops a redness or blue-gray discoloration over the pressure area.
- In dark-skinned people, the area may appear drier or the area will appear dark blue or black.

- The redness or discoloration does not go away within 30 minutes after the pressure has been relieved.
- The skin is not broken in Stage I.
- This stage is usually reversible if the area is detected promptly and pressure is relieved.
- Stage I may worsen rapidly.

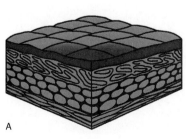

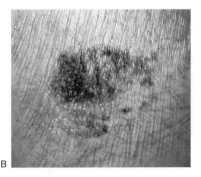

A   B

Figure 8-3   Development of a pressure ulcer—Stage I.

Stage II (Figure 8-4A, B):

- The skin is reddened, and there are abrasions, blisters, or a shallow crater at the site.
- The area around the breakdown site may also be reddened.
- The skin may or may not be broken.

- The epidermis alone or both the epidermis and the dermis may be involved.
- If this stage of development is neglected, further and deeper damage occurs.

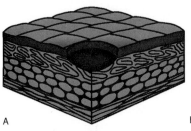
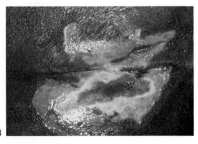

A   B

Figure 8-4   Development of a pressure ulcer—Stage II.

Stage III (Figure 8-5A, B):

- All the layers of the skin are destroyed, and a deep crater forms.

- The nurse documents the stage of the lesion using a commercial scale.

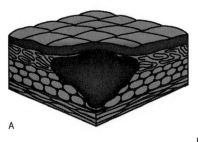
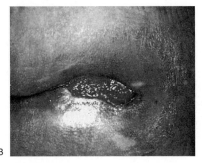

A

                                    B

Figure 8-5   Development of a pressure ulcer—Stage III.

Stage IV (Figure 8-6A, B):

- The ulcer extends through the skin and subcutaneous tissues.
- It may involve bone, muscle, and other structures.

- The patient will experience fluid loss.
- Patient is at great risk of infection.

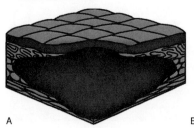
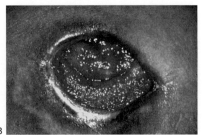

A   B

Figure 8-6   Development of a pressure ulcer—Stage IV.

Guidelines for Prevention of Pressure Ulcers

Nursing assistant actions are vital in identifying potential causes of breakdown and eliminating or minimizing them. The following care should be given:

- Change the patient's position at least every 2 hours. Some patients will require positioning more often. A major shift in position is required. When positioning a patient, be careful to avoid friction, such as sliding the patient over bedclothes or against equipment. Use lifting devices to avoid dragging. The care plan for each patient must be followed carefully. The turning schedule will be posted in the care plan and in the room.
- Encourage patients sitting in geri-chairs or wheelchairs to raise themselves frequently to relieve pressure, or assist patients to do so.
- Encourage proper nutrition and adequate intake of fluids. Breakdown occurs more readily and healing is delayed when the patient is poorly nourished. Proper nutrition may require tube feedings with enriched high-protein and high-vitamin supplements. Patients who are able to eat should be encouraged to do so. Adequate fluids are a requirement.
- Immediately remove feces or urine from the skin, because they are very irritating. Wash and dry the area immediately.
- Whenever giving personal care to patients, carefully inspect areas where pressure ulcers commonly form. Report any reddened areas immediately.
- Inspect skin daily and report the condition.
- Keep the skin clean and dry.

- Keep linen dry and free from wrinkles and hard objects such as crumbs and hairpins.
- Bathe patient frequently. Pay particular attention to potential pressure or friction areas. Avoid hot water and friction.
- Keep the skin supple and well lubricated with lotion. Do not massage directly on the site, and do not use alcohol. Apply moisturizers on dry skin by patting. Do not rub vigorously.
- Do not use lotion on broken skin.
- Separate body areas that are likely to rub together, especially over bony prominences, by using pillows or foam wedges according to the care plan.
- Use mechanical aids, such as foam padding, sheepskin, or an alternating-pressure mattress, to reduce pressure, friction, and shearing.
- Protect areas at risk, such as heels and elbows.
- Use a turning sheet to move dependent patients in bed.
- Elevate the head of the bed no higher than 30 degrees, to prevent a shearing effect on the tissues.
- Carry out range-of-motion exercises at least twice daily to encourage circulation.
- Check for improperly fitted or worn braces and restraints.
- Check nasogastric tubes and urinary catheters to be sure they are not a source of irritation. Keep the nasal and urinary openings clean and free of drainage. Check these areas frequently and carefully.
- Use sheepskin and foam cushions between patients and bottom linen, wheelchair backs, or wheelchair seats.
- For patients sitting in geri-chairs or wheelchairs, use foam, gel, or air cushions to reduce pressure on

buttocks and sacrum. Routinely check skin conditions.

• For patients in bed, relieve pressure on heels by supporting feet off the bed. Pad between legs when patient is on side.

• Report signs of infection, such as fever, odor, drainage, inflammation, or bleeding, to the nurse.

Nursing Assistant Actions When Skin Breakdown Occurs

• Perform the actions listed in the guidelines to prevent further breakdown.

• Follow the care plan exactly.

• Report indications of infection.

• Keep the area around the breakdown clean and dry.

• Assist with whirlpool baths, if ordered, to keep the area clean.

• The nurse or physician may perform other procedures to care for areas of skin breakdown.

• Encourage patients to participate in their own care.

• Attentive nursing care is essential in preventing additional skin breakdown. Remember that it is far easier to prevent pressure ulcers than to heal them.

Blood Circulation to Tissues

A major factor in preventing skin breakdown is ensuring adequate circulation to tissues:

• Position the patient correctly.

• Use mechanical aids.

• Give backrubs.

• Perform active or passive range-of-motion exercises.

Positioning

Positioning is used to relieve pressure as the patient's condition permits. Each position must be supported for comfort.

Patients with special problems require extra care when they are positioned in bed:

• Be sure the patient can breathe properly.

• Remember that a fractured hip is never rotated over the unaffected leg.

• If the patient had a stroke, elevate the weak arm to reduce edema.

• Always maintain proper body alignment.

• The patient with a recent stroke is turned on the unaffected side.

Chair Positioning

Proper chair positioning is essential to pressure ulcer prevention. This is one reason that the words "bedsore" and "decubitus ulcer" are dated and no longer acceptable or in widespread use. Both terms imply that the patient must be bedfast to experience skin breakdown, and this is not true. (*Decubitus* means lying down.) Pressure ulcers also can develop when the patient is in a chair, so attention to position, pressure relief, and frequent movement are important.

Stabilizing the patient's feet on the floor or wheelchair footrests is the first step to good chair positioning. Supporting the feet has an additional benefit, in that it keeps the patient from sliding forward in the wheelchair. For good posture and even weight distribution, the feet should be at a 90-degree angle to the lower legs. The lower legs should be at a 90-degree angle to the thighs. The thighs should be at a 90-degree angle to the torso. This is called the *90-90-90 position* (Figure 8-7), and it is key to pressure relief and good body mechanics when the patient is sitting in a chair or wheelchair.

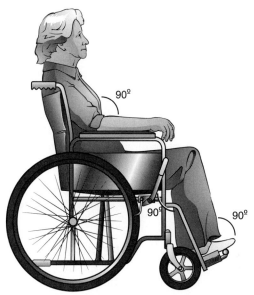

Figure 8-7   Good positioning begins with stabilizing the feet on the floor or wheelchair footrests. Position patients in the wheelchair and chair in the 90-90-90 position. This means that the feet are at a 90 degree angle to the lower legs. The lower legs are at a 90 degree angle to the thighs. The thighs are at a 90 degree angle to the torso. Additional benefits of this position are that it prevents sliding forward on the wheelchair seat and distributes weight and pressure evenly on the buttocks and upper legs.

Protecting the Feet

Bedfast patients are at very high risk of developing pressure ulcers on the feet and ankles. Patients with hip fractures are at great risk. The heels and ankles are at greatest risk of ulceration, although occasionally ulcers develop on the toes and the sides of the foot.

- Foot ulcers are easy to prevent by propping the calves on pillows positioned lengthwise. This suspends the heels over the surface of the bed, relieving all pressure.
- Follow the patient's care plan.

Other measures to prevent pressure ulcers on the feet and ankles are:

- Keep the skin well lubricated with lotion (avoid area between toes).
- Protect the feet from injury.
- Make sure the patient is wearing properly fitting footwear when out of bed.
  - The patient should always wear socks under shoes.
  - He or she should never ambulate barefoot or wearing only socks.
- Make sure bed linen is not too tight on the feet; use a bed cradle to keep the bedding away from the skin, if needed.
- Make sure footwear is not too tight; if footwear fits tightly, notify the nurse.

- Monitor the skin on the feet and ankles daily and report abnormalities promptly.

Burns

Whenever large sections of skin are destroyed, the body loses fluid and chemicals called electrolytes, and it becomes vulnerable to infection. Burns are a common cause of loss of large amounts of skin.

Classification

The temperature and length of exposure determine the severity of the burn. Prognosis is based on the extent of the burns. Burns are commonly classified as first-, second-, and third-degree. Burns may also be classified according to the depth of tissue involvement:

- First-degree burns (partial thickness) involve only the epidermis. The skin is pink to red, and there may be some temporary swelling and pain. There is usually no permanent damage or scarring.
- Second-degree burns (partial thickness) affect both epidermis and dermis. The color may vary from pink or red to white or tan. The burns cause blistering and pain and some scarring.
- Third-degree burns (full thickness) affect the epidermis, dermis, and subcutaneous tissue. The tissue is bright red to tan and brown, and the area is covered with a tough, leathery coat (eschar). There is no pain initially because nerve endings are destroyed. Later, pain and scarring will result.

When the epidermis, dermis, subcutaneous tissues, muscles, and bones are involved, the tissue appears blackened. Scarring will be extensive.

Nursing Assistant Care

- Report pain so that appropriate analgesics may be given.
- Maintain proper alignment.
- Use gentle positioning, as ordered, to prevent contractures.
- Encourage a high-protein diet.
- Carefully measure intake and output.
- Give emotional support and encouragement.
- Apply infection control rules.
- Apply the principles of standard precautions and wear gloves if contact with burned skin areas is likely.

PEDICULOSIS

Pediculosis is another term for lice. Three common types of lice are seen on patients in the United States:

- head lice (*pediculosis capitis*) —found on the head, scalp, and behind the ears
- body lice (*pediculosis corporis*, cooties) —found on the body and in clothing of infested people
- pubic lice (*pediculosis pubis*, crabs) —found in the pubic area; occasionally seen in underarm and eyebrow hair in humans

All three lice survive by sucking human blood. They are not found on birds, dogs, cats, farm animals, or other hosts. Lice on the skin tend to look like many, tiny red or brown scabs (Figure 8-8). Because they look like scabs, they may not be recognized as an abnormality. Study the appearance of the pictures in the text so you are able to recognize them.

Lice are tiny, so it is unlikely that you will see them moving about on the skin surface. They can survive only approximately 48 hours after separation from the human host. Hairs covering the louse's body can

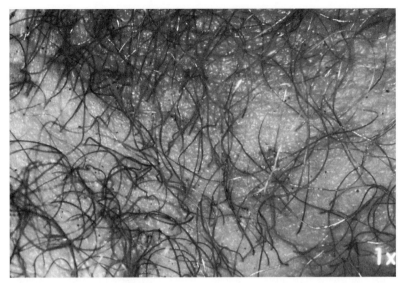

Figure 8-8 The tiny red-brown dots look like scabs, but are actually lice that are firmly attached to the skin. They are red-brown in color because they have recently consumed a blood meal.

pick up and send information to the insect about changes in the environment, such as body temperature and chemical changes within the host's body. The photos of most lice show a dark mass inside the abdomen. This is blood from a previously ingested meal. A louse that has not eaten recently is transparent in appearance. Lice cause most patients to complain of severe itching. Even if the patient does not complain, you will probably notice them scratching frequently and intensely. The itching is caused by lice feces, which are very irritating to the skin. Body lice and pubic lice are not found on animals. They are found only on humans.

Estimates are that more than 12 million people contract pubic lice in the United States annually. Approximately 20 million contract head lice each year. Treatment for head lice is believed to cost about $400 million annually.

Unfortunately, lice are hardy and adaptable, and have become resistant to many of the available treatments. Some of the home remedies, such as pouring gasoline on the scalp, hair, and body, have caused serious injuries and fatalities. Many of the treatment products cause complications in small children, frail elderly, pregnant women, persons with asthma and ragweed allergies, and persons with nonintact skin. Some people overtreat themselves and family members with over-the-counter products because the intense itching is not immediately relieved with treatment. The treatment products contain pesticides, and over time, these can cause complications related to product toxicity. Presence of the lice is of concern because they carry several serious diseases, including typhus and trench fever, which are not commonly seen in the U.S. and may not be recognized if a patient developed signs and symptoms. If not treated promptly and effectively, typhus can be fatal.

Body and pubic lice are commonly seen in, but not restricted to, unclean people who do not change their clothing regularly. The lice often hide in the seams of unwashed clothing. They deposit their nits in the soiled clothing, and occasionally on body hairs. Washing clothes in hot water and drying them in a hot dryer kills the lice. After infestation, the person can spread lice through direct contact or through clothing and bed linen. Lice are also transferred through sexual contact and other close personal contact. There are reports of the spread of pubic lice on toilet seats, but this is rare. Pubic lice live only on hairy parts of the body. They look like tiny crabs, and their legs are adapted to grasp the hair shart. They are most commonly seen on the pubic region, but occasionally are found in underarm hair, eyebrows, eyelashes, and head hair. Pubic lice deposit their nits on pubic hairs.

If lice are identified on a patient, a medicated cream or lotion must be applied. The patient will be in contact precautions for a brief period of time. All clothing and bed linen must be washed.

SCABIES

Another parasite contracted by humans is scabies. These parasites cause similar signs and symptoms, but the rash seems to follow the path of the blood vessels. Scabs and rashes on the skin are not a normal condition. Parasites are uncomfortable. Most are highly contagious, and some cause illness and infection. Scratching causes breaks in the skin integrity, which increases the risk of further breakdown and infection. Report any unusual rashes, scabs, or patient complaints of itching or scratching to the nurse for further assessment. Review Chapter 6 of this book and Units 12 and 38 of your text for additional information and pictures of parasites, head lice, and scabies.

DISORDERS OF THE RESPIRATORY SYSTEM

CHAPTER

9

Signs and symptoms that indicate problems with oxygen use and observations to report promptly to the nurse are listed in Table 9-1.

PATIENTS AT RISK OF POOR OXYGENATION

Hypoxemia is a condition in which there is insufficient oxygen in the blood. Patients who are immobile and those on bedrest have an increased risk of hypoxemia. When hypoxemia develops, immobility is a barrier to positive outcomes.

Checking capillary refill is a quick means of evaluating how well oxygen gets to body tissues. You may also use the pulse oximeter for monitoring patients with high-risk conditions.

UPPER RESPIRATORY INFECTIONS

An upper respiratory infection (URI) follows invasion of the upper respiratory organs by microbes. A common cold, which is caused by a virus, is an example of a URI. It is one of the most common illnesses found in people and usually is self-limiting.

Table 9-1 SIGNS AND SYMPTOMS OF INADEQUATE BREATHING

REPORT THE FOLLOWING SIGNS AND SYMPTOMS TO THE NURSE IMMEDIATELY

Movement in the chest is absent, minimal, or irregular.

Breathing movement appears to be in the abdomen, not the lungs.

Air movement cannot be detected by listening and feeling for breath sounds on your cheek and ear.

Respiratory rate is too slow or rapid.

Respirations are irregular, gasping, very deep, or shallow.

Respirations appear labored.

Patient is short of breath.

Patient's skin, lips, tongue, earlobes, mucous membranes, or nail beds are blue or gray.

Patient is short of breath and unable to speak at all or to speak in sentences.

Respirations are noisy.

Nasal flaring is present during inspiration.

The muscles below the ribs and/or above the clavicles retract inward during respiration.

You must take special note of and report the following:

- Dyspnea (difficult breathing)
- Changes in rate and rhythm of respiration
- Presence and character, color, and amount of respiratory secretions
- Cough
- Changes in skin color, such as pallor or cyanosis

URIs sometimes move down the chest and develop into bronchitis or even pneumonia.

PNEUMONIA

Pneumonia is a serious inflammation of the lungs. It can be caused by a variety of infectious organisms. Today most pneumonias, though serious and potentially life-threatening, respond favorably to antibiotic therapy.

CHRONIC OBSTRUCTIVE PULMONARY DISEASE

Chronic obstructive pulmonary disease (COPD) is also called chronic obstructive lung disease (COLD). This term refers to conditions that result in chronic blockage or obstruction of the respiratory system that is not reversible. Several conditions constitute COPD, including:

- Emphysema
- Chronic bronchitis
- Bronchiectasis

It can be very difficult to differentiate asthma from COPD, particularly in older patients.

ASTHMA

Asthma is a breathing disorder resulting from:

- Constriction of the muscles of the bronchioles.
- Swelling of the respiratory membranes.

- Production of large amounts of mucus that fill the narrowed passageways.

A person having an asthma attack has labored breathing and frequent coughing. An attack may result when the person contacts an allergen.

If a patient has known allergies (hypersensitivity to specific items), they should be marked in his or her health record.

CHRONIC BRONCHITIS

Chronic bronchitis is prolonged inflammation in the bronchi due to infection or irritants. Signs and symptoms include:

- Swollen and red bronchial tissues, resulting in narrowed bronchial passageways
- Persistent cough
- Sputum production
- Respiratory distress

EMPHYSEMA

Emphysema develops after chronic obstruction of the air flow to the alveoli. The patient can bring air into the lungs, but it becomes more difficult to expel air from the lungs. As a result, there is less and less room for air to reenter. There is no sputum production. However, patients with emphysema are at high risk of developing pneumonia. This condition also causes the heart to work harder. The most common sign of respiratory problems in a patient with emphysema is headache, which is caused by increasing carbon dioxide levels in the blood. Other signs and symptoms of emphysema are:

- Fatigue
- Chronic oxygen deprivation
- Difficulty breathing
- Loss of appetite and weight loss

General Care

The care of patients with COPD includes:

- Assisting with proper breathing techniques, such as pursed-lip breathing
- Encouraging breathing exercises
- Positioning to improve ventilation
- Assisting with postural drainage (this therapy is not commonly used for emphysema)
- Providing care during low-flow oxygen therapy
- Paying attention to nutrition and fluid intake
- Treating infections with antibiotics and drugs to loosen and thin respiratory secretions
- Encouraging fluid intake
- Taking annual flu shots and the pneumonia vaccine at the frequency specified by the health care provider
- Encouraging patients to avoid crowds, especially during the flu season
- Encouraging patients not to smoke
- Wearing gloves if your hands may contact the patient's respiratory secretions
- Wearing a gown, goggles, or face shield, and a surgical mask if the patient is coughing and spraying respiratory secretions into the air

SURGICAL CONDITIONS

Most respiratory problems are not treated with surgery. However, several problems require surgical correction to ensure uninterrupted air flow.

Tracheostomy

A tracheostomy is done for some patients who have had head and neck surgery, and some victims of serious trauma. It may also be done for patients who need a ventilator to support their breathing for a long time or need suctioning to clear airway secretions.

A tracheostomy may be temporary or permanent. The external opening on the skin surface is the stoma. Caring for the tracheostomy is the nurse's responsibility. Notify him or her immediately if the ties are loose or any part of the device comes apart or is removed. The ties can be too tight, too. You should be able to slide your finger underneath the tie on either side of the neck. If you cannot, it is too tight, and you need to notify the nurse immediately.

MALIGNANCIES

Malignant tumors can develop in any part of the respiratory tract. Lung cancers are treated by surgery, radiation, chemotherapy, or a combination of all three therapies.

Cancer of the Larynx

Cancer of the larynx may require removal of the larynx, resulting in the loss of the voice. The patient breathes through a stoma, an artificial opening in the neck and trachea. Although it may look like a regular tracheostomy, it is very different. If you are caring for a patient with a stoma, you must know whether it is a tracheostomy stoma or a laryngectomy stoma. If the patient has a tracheostomy, the passageway from the mouth and nose through the trachea remains intact. The patient can still smell odors, blow his or her nose, and suck on a straw. If a patient has had a laryngectomy, the larynx (voice box) has been removed. The upper airway is no longer connected to the trachea. The patient will not be able to smell, blow his or her nose, whistle, gargle, or suck on a straw.

Postsurgical care is given in the acute care hospital. At this time, writing is the major form of communication available to such patients. Later, the patient may be taught new ways to speak through esophageal speech or electronic speech.

Patients with laryngectomies need patience and understanding from all health care providers. A difficult psychological adjustment must be made by the patient. The loss of one's voice requires an adjustment similar to that experienced when grieving for the loss of a loved one. Expect periods of depression, anger, and hostility.

Caring for a Patient with a Tracheostomy or Laryngectomy Stoma

Humidified oxygen may be administered to patients with a tracheostomy. The stoma provides a direct passageway into the lungs. Because of this:

- Some patients wear a mask similar to a surgical mask over the opening. The risk of inhaling a foreign particle is greatly increased. Inhaling small objects or water (such as during a shower) can cause serious complications.
- Check with the nurse or care plan for precautions to take when showering the patient.
- *Avoid getting powder, lint, dust, water, or other objects near or in the stoma. Likewise, the opening in the neck provides an open pathway for bacteria to enter, causing infection.*
- *Use standard precautions and frequent hand washing when caring for a patient with a stoma. Secretions may be expelled from the stoma when the patient coughs. The patient has no control over this.*
- *If the patient is expelling secretions, you will also need to wear a gown, mask, and eye protection when caring for him or her.*

Chest Tubes

Chest tube insertion is almost always an emergency procedure. Chest drainage is not done for minor problems. Tubes are inserted only if a condition is life-threatening. It is not done for patients who have blood clotting problems. Chest tubes are inserted to treat:

- *pneumothorax,* or an air leak from the lung into the chest cavity, which may occur spontaneously, although this is not as common as other causes.
- *hemothorax,* or bleeding into the chest.
- *empyema,* which is pus in the chest or a lung abscess.

The tubes are used to remove free air from the chest cavity. This problem results from trauma, injuries, and some medical conditions. When a lung collapses, the pressure change makes breathing very difficult. The patient may complain of feeling like an elephant is standing on his or her chest. Removing fluids from the chest through the tube enables the lung to reinflate. Chest tubes also:

- drain bloody fluid from the chest after surgery (usually a pneumothorax or hemothorax that develops after surgery or from trauma to the chest).
- enable air to escape if there is a leak at the suture line after lung surgery.
- treat *pleural effusion,* a condition that occurs when fluid collects around the lungs in patients with cancer.

Caring for a Patient with a Chest Tube

The chest tube is attached to a drain of some sort. The nurse will manage the system. To help monitor and care for the patient:

- Make sure that nothing pulls on the tube that comes out of the chest.
- Position the drainage system in an upright position, below the level of the heart at all times.
- Reposition the patient every 2 hours or as instructed.
- Make sure the chest tube is never twisted, kinked, or obstructed.
- Coil the tubing that connects the chest tube to the drain on the bed the same way you would position tubing for a Foley catheter.
- If the drain is connected to a vacuum regulator, do not disconnect it.
- Seat the patient in a chair to keep him mobile, as permitted.
- Always have oxygen, suction, and emergency equipment set up at the bedside. Never remove these items.

Notify the nurse if the:

- Vital signs change
- Pulse oximeter alarm sounds
- Dressing on the chest wall is loose
- Color or amount of drainage from the chest tube changes
- Patient coughs up blood
- Patient becomes short of breath or cyanotic
- Patient develops new swelling on the torso, neck, or face that "crackles" when touched
- Tube comes out

Oxygen Therapy

Oxygen is often ordered by the physician. Remember that when oxygen is in use, special precautions are required to prevent fires and to administer the oxygen safely.

Special safety measures must be emphasized in areas where oxygen is being used:

- *Be certain that there are no open flames and that no one smokes or has matches.*
- *Post "no smoking" or "oxygen-in-use" signs.*

Hospitals have oxygen piped from wall units directly into the patient's room. In some cases, the oxygen source is a tank that is brought to the patient's room when therapy is ordered. The amount of oxygen (rate of flow measured in liters) is ordered by the physician. If you are responsible for setting up or maintaining any type of oxygen delivery system, *never modify an oxygen system to make the parts fit together. If you cannot connect it readily, seek further help.*

Caring for a Patient Receiving Oxygen Therapy

The care plan may instruct you to:

- Elevate the head of the bed when the patient is receiving oxygen. This will make it easier to breathe.
- Patients using oxygen masks cannot eat meals while wearing the mask. The physician may order a nasal cannula at mealtime. Follow the instructions on the care plan or critical pathway for patient care measures.

Being unable to breathe is very frightening. Patients who are receiving oxygen may need:

- Reassurance and emotional support.
- Check on the patient frequently and spend as much time in the room as possible. Difficult breathing makes it hard to talk. The patient may be unable to hold a normal conversation. Just being with the patient without talking is very reassuring.
- If the patient is having trouble breathing, try to ask questions that can be answered yes or no.

You will care for patients using different devices for the administration of oxygen. Carefully check the skin under the device.

- Make sure that it does not become red or irritated from the elastic that holds it in place. Report any skin problems to the nurse.
- Offer extra liquids to drink.

Patients also need:

- Frequent care of the mouth, lips, and nose. The patient may need care of the mucous membranes every few hours. Oxygen causes the mucous membranes to dry out, which is very uncomfortable. You may be instructed to wipe the nostrils with a cotton applicator moistened with normal saline. Mouth care is usually given with a sponge-tipped applicator or lemon-glycerine swab. Keep the patient's lips moist with water-soluble lubricant or lip balm.
- Sometimes patients feel warm and will perspire heavily. Extra bathing and linen changes may be necessary. You may need to adjust the temperature in the room and help the patient change into a hospital gown. Cover him or her with a sheet. The care plan or critical pathway will provide information on patient preferences and needs.

When caring for a patient using oxygen, you should:

- Wear gloves and apply the principles of standard precautions if contact with the patient's oral or nasal secretions is likely.
- Know the flow rate that was ordered and set for your patient.
- Be able to read the flowmeter for the rate of oxygen delivery if instructed to check the rate by the nurse.
- Notify the nurse immediately if there is a change in the flow rate.

- Check that the tubing is not obstructed in any way that would prevent oxygen from reaching the patient.
- Check for proper position of the catheter, cannula, or mask and that the elastic band around the head is snug but not constricting.
- Use a portable tank for patient transport to other areas of the hospital.
- Do not remove the oxygen without the RCP's or RN's permission.

If a tank is used as the source of oxygen, be sure that:

- There is sufficient oxygen in the tank. Check the gauge each time you visit the patient.
- The oxygen is on.
- An additional tank is available to exchange for the tank in use when it is empty.
- Empty tanks are marked and stored according to facility policy.
- The tank is upright and securely chained to the wall, carrier, or in the stand.

Humidifiers

In some facilities, a humidifier is attached to the oxygen administration equipment if the patient's flow exceeds 5 liters.

Sterile distilled water is always used in the humidifier. Avoid tap water. Inhalation of tap water is associated with an increased incidence of Legionnaires' disease. The water level in the humidifier should always be at or above the "minimum fill" line on the bottle.

METHODS OF OXYGEN DELIVERY

Oxygen may be delivered to the patient by several methods. The same basic care is required for each method, with minor modifications.

- *Nasal cannula:* Delivery of oxygen by nasal cannula is the most common method used today. The oxygen is delivered through a tube that has two small plastic prongs. The prongs are placed at the entrance to the patient's nose. A strap around the patient's head holds the prongs in place.
  - Make sure the strap is secure but not too tight.
  - Check for signs of irritation where the prongs touch the patient's nose.
  - Check that mucus has not blocked the prong openings. Clean if necessary.
  - Make sure the cannula is stored when not in use in such a way that it is not contaminated.

- *Mask:* The oxygen mask is a cup-like mask held in place by straps around the head. The oxygen mask fits over the patient's nose, mouth, and chin. Several kinds of face masks are used, depending on the patient's oxygen needs. A special mask fits over a tracheostomy. Using an oxygen mask is necessary when high liter flows of oxygen are ordered. Masks may also be used for individuals who breathe through their mouths.

  A mask is never used with flows under 5 liters because it will cause rebreathing of exhaled carbon dioxide and has a smothering effect.

  Some masks have inflatable bags at the bottom. The combination of bag and mask increases the amount of oxygen delivered to the patient. The bag should be inflated at all times. Notify the nurse if the bag collapses more than halfway during inspiration.

Oxygen Concentrator

An oxygen concentrator takes in room air and removes impurities and gases other than oxygen, allowing the oxygen to become concentrated in the unit. The air delivered to the patient from the concentrator is more than 90% oxygen. It is delivered by tubing attached to a nasal cannula. The flow rate is usually 2 liters per minute (L/min).

General Oxygen Concentrator Precautions

Follow these precautions when a concentrator is used to supply oxygen to a patient:

- Place concentrator at least 5 feet away from any heat source and at least 4 inches from the wall.
- Smoking is not permitted in the same room.
- Be sure the unit is plugged in and grounded.
- Do not use an extension cord with the concentrator.
- Never change the flowmeter setting.
- Notify the nurse if the alarm sounds.
- A mask is not used with a concentrator because the exhaled carbon dioxide cannot be expelled with low liter flows of oxygen.
- Wipe cannula daily with a damp cloth (do not use alcohol- or oil-based products). Change according to facility policy.
- Clean concentrator surfaces using a damp cloth only.
- Remove the filter weekly. Wash in warm soapy water, rinse, squeeze dry, and replace.

Liquid Oxygen

Oxygen also comes in a canister in liquid form.

Safety Precautions for Liquid Oxygen:

Liquid oxygen is nontoxic, but it will cause severe burns on direct contact.

- *Avoid opening, touching, or spilling the container.*
- *If your skin or clothing contacts the liquid oxygen, flush with a large amount of water.*
- *Follow all safety precautions for preventing sparks and fires.*
- *Never seal the cap or vent port on the liquid oxygen.*
- *If a bottle falls or tips, remove the patient from the room and close the door. Notify the nurse promptly.*

RESPIRATORY POSITIONS

Position the patient in:
- High Fowler's position
- Orthopneic position
- Tripod position

The tripod position is a good alternative to improve ventilation. The patient sits as upright as possible and leans slightly forward, supporting him- or herself with the forearms. This position makes the thorax larger on inspiration, enabling the patient to inhale more air.
- Allow the patient to sit on the side of the bed.
- Support the legs.
- The patient can lean across an overbed table, if desired.

INCENTIVE SPIROMETER

The physician may write orders for use of an incentive spirometer to help the lungs expand fully. This prevents atelectasis (collapse of the alveoli) and also helps prevent pneumonia.

This procedure may be carried out with the patient in bed, with head and shoulders well supported, if permitted. The procedure is usually taught before surgery.

Nursing Assistant Responsibilities

- Observe the patient for correctness of procedure.
- Advise the patient not to take in too many deep breaths in a row, which will cause dizziness.
- Encourage the patient to cough and clear respiratory passages.
- Report to the nurse if the patient seems overly fatigued during the procedure.
- Carefully observe and report any unusual responses such as pain, dizziness, or throat and airway irritation.
- When the patient has completed the pulmonary exercise, wash the mouthpiece in warm water, dry it, replace it in the plastic bag, and leave it at the bedside.
- Patients should be praised for their efforts. Many times this encourages greater effort the next time the incentive spirometer is used.

OTHER TECHNIQUES

Continuous Positive Airway Pressure (CPAP)

Some patients stop breathing periodically while they sleep. This condition is called sleep apnea. Treatment in many cases is with a CPAP device that delivers pressure to the airway while the patient sleeps; this pressure holds the airway open.

Nursing Assistant Responsibilities

- Remind the patient to wash and dry his or her face thoroughly before putting on the mask.
- Monitor the patient while he or she is connected to a CPAP machine.
- Make sure the mask is comfortable.

- Avoid leaks around the top. If this happens, you can adjust the mask to see if you can reduce the leak. On the other hand, if the mask is too tight, the patient may feel pain, or there may be redness or skin breakdown on the nose.
- If the patient complains of excessive dryness, inform the nurse.
- Avoid petrolatum products with respiratory devices.
- If a patient swallows a lot of air from the mask, belches frequently, and feels pressure in the abdomen, elevate the head of the bed.
- Wash the mask in soap and water each morning.
- Store the dry mask in a clean plastic bag until use at bedtime.

COLLECTING A SPUTUM SPECIMEN

You may need to collect a sputum specimen from the patient. Sputum is matter that is brought up (expectorated) from the lungs. A culture of the specimen identifies the cause of an infection.

You must be sure that the specimen comes from the lungs and is not saliva from the mouth.

If the patient cannot expectorate sputum, suctioning may be needed to obtain the specimen. (The nurse performs this procedure.) It is easier to collect the specimen when the patient wakes up in the morning and after taking two or three deep breaths.

DISORDERS OF THE CARDIOVASCULAR SYSTEM

CARDIOVASCULAR SYSTEM

Observations to report in patients with disorders of the cardiovascular system are:

- Color change, pallor or cyanosis, redness
- Skin is cool to touch
- Skin is hot to touch
- Changes in pulse rate or rhythm
- Changes in blood pressure
- Edema
- Disorientation

PERIPHERAL VASCULAR DISEASES

Peripheral vascular diseases that affect the arteries diminish the flow of blood to the extremities. Tissues through which the narrowed arteries pass may not get the nourishment they need. Areas affected are the extremities: arms, legs, and brain.

Nursing Assistant Responsibilities

- Increasing local circulation
  - Positioning and specific prescribed exercises can promote arterial flow and venous return.
  - Nothing that would hamper the patient's circulation is permitted.
- Preventing injuries that heal poorly

Guidelines for Caring for Patients with Peripheral Vascular Disease

- Elevate the feet when the patient is sitting in a chair for a long time.

When the feet are not elevated, make sure that the patient's feet are flat on the floor. If they are not, support the feet with a footstool. Discourage the patient from crossing the legs when sitting.

- Discourage smoking—it interferes with circulation.
- Avoid using the knee gatch of the bed.
- Avoid using heating pads or hot water bottles. The patient may not feel temperatures that are too hot.
- Maintain body warmth. Make sure the patient has warm clothes, including well-fitting socks. Provide blankets for the bed.
- Prevent injury to the feet:
  - Instruct the patient to wear shoes and socks when out of bed.
  - Check to see that the shoes are in good repair and that they fit well. Inform the nurse if footwear is too tight.
  - Avoid pressure to the legs and feet from any source.
- Inspect the feet carefully when you bathe the patient or if the patient complains of any discomfort in the feet. Promptly report any signs of inflammation, injury, or circulatory problems:
  - Broken skin
  - Color change—redness, whiteness, or cyanosis
  - Heat or coldness
  - Cracking between toes
  - Corns or calluses

- Swelling
- Pain
- Loss of sensation or function
- Drainage
- Bathe the feet regularly.
  - Dry thoroughly and gently between the toes.
  - Use a moisturizing lotion on the feet and legs if the skin is dry.
- Do not cut the toenails of patients with peripheral vascular disease. Avoid using sharp objects such as a nail file on the toes.
- Make sure bed linen is not too tight on the feet. Use a bed cradle, if ordered.
- Check the skin under support hose regularly; remove the hose periodically, according to the plan of care.
- Prop the patient's calves on pillows that are positioned lengthwise so that the heels are elevated from the surface of the bed, or position the patient so that the heels hang over the end of the mattress with the soles of the feet against a footboard. Do not position the pillow widthwise under the calves. Heel protectors are excellent for preventing friction and shearing, but they do not prevent pressure on the heels. Other devices are available to keep the heels away from the surface of the bed to relieve pressure. Follow the care plan and the nurse's instructions.
- Make sure the feet are supported on footrests when the patient is using the wheelchair; avoid dragging them across the floor.

Varicose Veins

- Report the following:
  - Signs of rash, irritation, or breakdown
  - Pain or aching in the legs
  - Signs of inflammation (warmth and redness)
- Follow the care plan.
- Keep the feet clean and dry.
- Avoid injury.
- Apply antiembolism hose, if ordered.
- *Never rub or massage the area of a varicose vein.*

Transient Ischemic Attack

Transient ischemic attack (TIA) is a temporary interruption of the blood flow to part of the brain. The patient may experience:

- Weakness or paralysis of any extremity or the face
- Vision problems
- Difficulty with speech
- Difficulty with swallowing

These symptoms come on quickly and may last from just a few minutes to 24 hours. There are no permanent effects. However, a TIA is usually a warning that a stroke will occur at some time.

If a patient has any of the symptoms listed, report them to the nurse immediately.

HEART CONDITIONS

Heart disease may sometimes be due to an infection, but usually it develops because of changes in the blood vessels. As the openings of the blood vessels become smaller, the heart must work harder and harder to do its job of pumping the blood to the body.

Angina Pectoris

Angina pectoris is known as cardiac "pain of effort." The coronary arteries are the blood vessels that nourish the heart. These vessels often are the site of atherosclerotic changes. In an angina attack, the vessels are unable to carry enough blood to meet the heart's demand for oxygen.

Factors that precipitate (bring on) an attack include:

- Exertion
- Heavy eating
- Emotional stress

The signs and symptoms of angina pectoris that you should immediately report include:

- Pain when exercising or under stress. Stress causes a need for an immediate increase in coronary circulation. The pain is described as dull, with increasing intensity. It is usually centered under the breastbone (sternum), spreading to the left arm and up into the neck.
- Pale or flushed face.
- Patient who is freely perspiring.

Signs and symptoms may differ from one individual to another, but the symptoms are usually the same each time a person experiences an attack. You may assist the patient who has angina pectoris by:

- Helping the patient to avoid unnecessary emotional or physical stress
- Encouraging the patient not to smoke
- Reporting any signs or symptoms of an attack to the nurse at once

Myocardial Infarction (Coronary Heart Attack)

The term myocardial infarction (MI), or heart attack, refers to a period in which the heart suddenly cannot function properly. There are different kinds of heart attacks, which differ in severity and prognosis (expected outcome). An acute MI occurs when the coronary arteries, which nourish the heart, are blocked. Part of the heart muscle supplied by these vessels becomes ischemic (loses its blood supply). Unless circulation is restored quickly, the cells die (infarction). If too much tissue dies, the person cannot survive.

Signs and Symptoms

The signs and symptoms of a heart attack include:

- Pain—may resemble severe indigestion. It is often described as "crushing" chest pain that radiates to the jaw and left arm.
- Nausea/vomiting.
- Irregular pulse and respiration.
- Perspiration (diaphoresis).
- Feelings of anxiety and weakness.
- Indications of shock, which include drop in blood pressure and pallor.
- Shortness of breath.
- Syncope (fainting).
- Restlessness.
- Cyanosis or gray color of skin, nailbeds, or mucous membrane.

The signs and symptoms of a heart attack vary with the individual. The pain may be located in the chest in some patients and may radiate to the jaw or either arm. If a patient has chest pain combined with any other signs or symptoms, he or she should be evaluated by a health care professional. Have the patient stop any activity immediately and assume a comfortable position.

Stay with the patient and call for assistance.

Immediate treatment has saved many people. The treatment is directed toward:

- Relieving the pain
- Reducing heart activity
- Altering the clotting ability of the blood
- Administering drugs to dissolve the clot

Nursing Care

Nursing care supports the therapy ordered. Special attention must be given to:

- Noting signs of a recurrence and reporting immediately to the nurse
- Watching for bleeding and reporting immediately
- Assisting with activities of daily living
- Monitoring vital signs

Congestive Heart Failure

Congestive heart failure (CHF) got its name because of *failure* of the *heart* to pump efficiently, which results in *congestion* of the lungs. The heart tries to compensate for the problem, but this worsens the condition.

Signs and Symptoms

The signs and symptoms are the result of the heart being unable to pump the blood with sufficient force.

- Hemoptysis (spitting up blood), cough
- Orthopnea (difficulty in breathing unless sitting upright) or dyspnea
- Ascites (fluid collecting in the abdomen)
- Prominent neck veins, fatigue
- Hypoxia (inadequate oxygen levels), confusion
- Edema (swelling) that is most common in the abdomen, ankles, and fingers
- Congestion, fluid accumulation in the lungs
- Waking up at night with breathlessness, inability to lie flat
- Cyanosis, irregular and rapid pulse
- High blood pressure, palpitations
- Liver or kidney malfunction

Nursing Assistant Responsibilities

- Serve a low-sodium diet.
- Restrict fluids, if ordered.
- Monitor intake and output.
- Weigh patient daily to monitor level of fluid retention.
- Monitor apical pulse and observing for pulse deficit.
- Monitor vital signs.
- Position patient in orthopneic position or high Fowler's supported by pillows, or supported in a chair.
- Change position frequently but slowly.
- Keep the weight of the bedding off the toes.
- Apply elasticized stockings or TED hose. Remove and reapply every 4 hours, or as specified on the care plan.
- Check circulation; the skin should be normal in color and warm.
- Assist with activities of daily living as needed. If complete bathing is tiring, give partial baths. Monitor the skin for breakdown.
- Allow the patient to be as independent with bathing as possible, if permitted.
- Check the patient frequently while he or she is bathing. Be prepared to take over and complete the bath if the patient becomes short of breath or too tired.
- Provide special mouth care, if needed.
- Provide a bedside commode for elimination.
- Encourage adequate nutrition. Provide small, easily digested meals.
- Assist in feeding the patient, if needed.
- Keep the feet elevated when up in the chair or wheelchair.
- Encourage regular rest periods throughout the day.
- Assist with exercise, as specified on the care plan.

Heart Block

Heart block is a condition that develops due to interference in the electrical current through the heart. An electronic device called a pacemaker is implanted that signals the heart to contract.

When caring for a patient who has a pacemaker:

- Count and record the pulse rate.
- Report any irregularities or changes below the present rate.
- Report any discoloration over the implant site.
- Report hiccupping, because this may indicate problems.
- Keep the patient away from microwave ovens and cellular phones, because they may disrupt the function of the pacemaker.

BLOOD ABNORMALITIES

Blood abnormalities are often called *blood dyscrasias*.

Anemia

Anemia is a condition that results from a decrease in the quantity or quality of red blood cells.

Leukemia

Leukemia is sometimes called cancer of the blood. The causes of the many forms of leukemia are not known. This disease may strike young or old. The number of white blood cells increases, but the white blood cells are immature and of poor quality. The number of erythrocytes and platelets decreases. Patients with leukemia are highly susceptible to infection. During the course of the disease, even minor trauma can cause bleeding.

Special Care

Patients who have leukemia or anemia require special care. You must:

- Check vital signs.
- Encourage rest and a good diet.
- Handle the patient very gently.
- Give special mouth care, because the mouth and tongue become sensitive. Report mouth sores to the nurse.
- Be sure to report any signs of bleeding, such as bruises or discolorations, because further blood loss makes the condition worse.
- Keep patient warm.
- Protect patient from falls that may result from dizziness or weakness.
- Change the patient's position often, at least every 2 hours.
- Provide emotional support.

DISORDERS OF THE MUSCULOSKELETAL SYSTEM

COMMON CONDITIONS

Many conditions can affect the bones, muscles, tendons, ligaments, and joints. Often, when one of these structures is diseased or injured, the surrounding tissues are also involved.

Bursitis

Bursae are small sacs of fluid located around joints. They help to reduce friction when muscles move. At times, the bursae can become inflamed, and the tissues around a joint may become painful. This condition is known as bursitis.

Arthritis

The term arthritis means inflammation of the joints. It may develop following an acute injury, or it may be chronic and progressive. The most common forms of chronic arthritis are:

1. *Rheumatoid arthritis (RA).* This affects the joint tissues and joint lining and can affect any other body system. It is a serious form of arthritis that can occur in persons of any age. Although the cause is not known, it is believed to be an autoimmune response. RA has exacerbations and remissions. The involved joints may feel hot to the touch. The condition causes reduced joint function and deformities.

2. *Osteoarthritic joint disease (OJD)* or *degenerative joint disease (DJD)* affects the cartilage covering the ends of the bones that form a joint. Cartilage breaks down, and the ends of the bones rub together, causing pain and deformity. The weight-bearing joints are most often affected. The most common symptom of osteoarthritis is pain. Other symptoms include limited ability to move and stiffness, particularly upon arising in the morning. Stiffness also may occur after strenuous exercise or physical overactivity. In some individuals, an audible grating sound can be heard in the joints during movement. Osteoarthritis may cause redness and swelling in the joints.

3. *Gout (gouty arthritis)* is a metabolic disease that can be severely disabling. It is caused by increased uric acid, which deposits in the joints, causing pain. It can occur in any joint but is most common in the feet and legs. The first symptom of illness is usually sudden onset of pain in the big toe with no history of injury. Gout is marked by constant pain, tenderness, and swelling in the joints. Other body systems may be affected in this stage. Dietary restrictions are used to reduce the uric acid level in the blood. The dietitian will plan a diet that restricts the amount of red meat and foods rich in purines.

Nursing Assistant's Role

Arthritis can cause mild discomfort to severe deformities and disability.

Patients with arthritis are at high risk of contractures.

- If permitted by your facility, place patients with this condition in the prone position periodically to reduce the risk of contractures of the hips and knees.
- Avoid placing pillows under the knees or elevating the knee area of the bed.
- Use a small, flat pillow under the head and neck.
- Perform range of motion as ordered.
- Be very gentle.
- Avoid moving joints past the point of resistance.

Osteoporosis

Osteoporosis is a metabolic disorder of the bones. It is most common in elderly females but can occur in males. Bone mass is lost, causing bones to appear porous and spongy. Consequently, affected bones are at very high risk for fracture. Fractures can occur spontaneously, such as when the patient is walking. They can also occur when the patient is moved or turned in bed or during transfers. Compression fractures are common.

Treatment

The goals of treatment are to:

- Prevent further fractures and control pain.
- Provide gentle range-of-motion and other exercises.
- Splints, braces, and other devices may be ordered.

You must handle the patient very gently. If you are assigned to perform range-of-motion exercises, do so slowly and carefully. Avoid stretching the joint past the point of resistance. Use a mechanical lift for transfers whenever possible. This is less traumatic

than pulling on the patient. Make sure you have extra help for all procedures in which you will be moving or positioning the patient. Follow the care plan exactly.

Bisphosphonates are a class of medications that are a common treatment for persons with osteoporosis and other bone disorders. Although the drugs have proven effective, their use is not without risk. Patients taking drugs in this category have specific requirements for eating, drinking, and maintaining an upright position. If you are caring for a patient who is taking a bisphosphonate drug, the care plan will list special precautions, times when meals and fluid schedules must be altered. Drugs in this category are usually given immediately upon arising for the day, and at least 30 minutes to two hours before or after eating. The instructions vary slightly from one drug to the next. Some foods, such as calcium products and antacid medications, are withheld when the drug is given. The patient is required to sit or stand for a period of time (usually 30 minutes) following medication administration. Preventing dehydration is very important. The patient must drink a full glass (8 ounces or more) of fluid when the drug is given, and intake and output monitoring is often ordered. Follow the care plan instructions very carefully. The nurse and the care plan will provide information about special monitoring.

Fibromyalgia

Fibromyalgia is a common chronic pain syndrome for which there is no known cause or cure. It affects more women than men. The pain is described as either a general soreness or a gnawing ache, and stiffness is usually worst in the morning. The

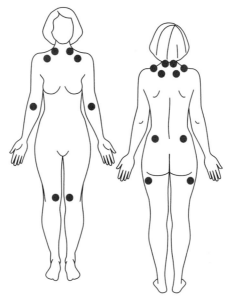

Figure 11-1 The patient must have pain at 11 of 18 specific areas for a diagnosis of fibromyalgia to be made.

condition can interfere with the patient's quality of life and daily activities.

Signs and Symptoms

Signs and symptoms of fibromyalgia are:

- Pain and stiffness
- Feeling abnormally tired
- Waking up tired
- Pain upon touch in certain areas of the body (Figure 11-1).

Fractures

A fracture is any break in the continuity of bone (Figure 11-2). Falls are the most common cause of fractures.

Signs and Symptoms

Signs and symptoms of fractures will vary with the type of fracture and location. Fractures are painful conditions. Movement is limited, or the patient will be unable to move the injured area. The skin surrounding the fracture may

appear deformed. Edema is common. Ecchymosis, or bruising, may occur. Some parts of the body, such as the area over the femur, are very vascular. They bleed readily under the skin. An ecchymosis the size of an adult's fist over the femur indicates loss of approximately one pint of blood.

Treatment

A new fracture is usually treated in the hospital emergency department. Admission for surgical correction of the fracture may be necessary. The immediate goals of care are to:

- Control pain
- Prevent complications of immobility
- Prevent or reduce edema
- Keep the fracture in good alignment
- Keep the fractured extremity immobile

Fractures of any kind are treated by keeping the part that is injured

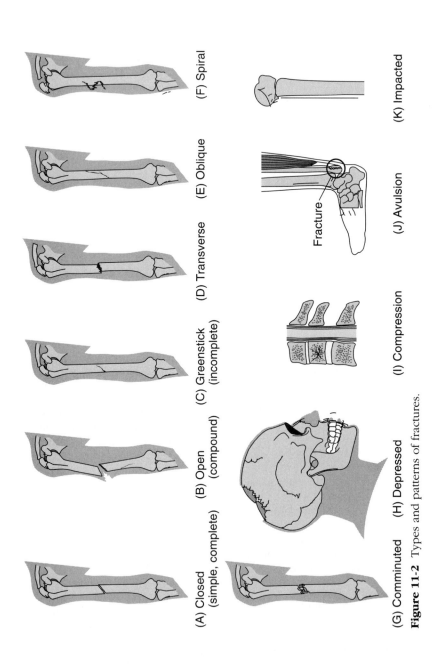

(A) Closed (simple, complete) (B) Open (compound) (C) Greenstick (incomplete) (D) Transverse (E) Oblique (F) Spiral

(G) Comminuted (H) Depressed (I) Compression (J) Avulsion (K) Impacted

Fracture

Figure 11-2 Types and patterns of fractures.

immobilized in proper position until healing takes place.

Care of Patients with Casts

Special care for the newly casted patient includes:

- Supporting the cast and body in good alignment with pillows covered by cloth pillowcases, and keeping the cast uncovered.
- You may be instructed to elevate the casted extremity on a pillow. When positioning a patient with a leg cast, elevate the foot higher than the hip. For an arm in a cast, the fingers should be higher than the elbow. Avoid placing the cast on a flat surface. Avoid placing anything plastic under a wet cast. Check the skin distal to the cast frequently for signs of poor circulation.
- Turning the patient frequently to permit air circulation to all parts of the cast. Maintain support. Use the palm of the hand, not fingers, to support the wet cast.
- Avoid positioning the cast against the footboard or side rail. Leaving the cast open to air until it dries is best. If the patient is cold, cover the cast loosely with a sheet. Avoid tucking the sheet under the mattress. A bed cradle may be used, if necessary. The greatest area of heat loss is the head. Covering the upper body and back and top of the head with a blanket may help keep the patient warm.
- Closely observing the uncasted areas of the extremities, such as the fingers and toes, for signs of decreased circulation. Report coldness, cyanosis, swelling, increased pain, numbness, or tingling immediately.
- Closely observing skin areas around the cast edges for signs of irritation. Rough edges should be covered with adhesive strips to prevent skin irritation.

Recall the following list of reportables when checking the patient:

- C = color
- M = motion
- E = edema
- T = temperature

Special Care after Cast Is Dry

After the cast has completely dried:

- Turn the patient to the noncasted side. This is particularly important in moving a patient with a body cast (spica cast) because turning to the casted side may crack the cast.
- Always support the cast when turning or moving the patient.
- Encourage use of an overhead bar, known as a trapeze, to assist the patient in helping him- or herself.
- Tape edges of casts to prevent pressure and abrasive areas, if edges were not covered when the cast was applied.
- Use plastic to protect cast edges that are near the genitals and buttocks, to help prevent soiling during toileting.

Changes that may occur after the cast dries that indicate infection or ulceration under the cast are:

- Odor from the cast
- Drainage through the cast

The care plan may instruct you to keep the casted extremity elevated, to prevent edema. A sling may be used to elevate an arm cast when the patient is out of bed. A wheelchair with an elevated leg rest is used for patients with leg casts. Cover the cast with plastic during bathing. Keep small objects from getting inside the cast. The patient may complain of an itching sensation under the cast. Discourage him or her from placing objects down the cast to scratch. This could cause a skin injury and infection. Report complaints of itching to the nurse.

Care of Patients in Traction

- Review the correct placement of straps and weights with the therapist or nurse.
- Get instructions for moving the patient up in bed and turning to the sides, as ordered.
- Avoid moving, dropping, or releasing the weights. They should not touch the bed, swing back and forth freely, or rest on any object or surface. The water bag or weight hangs still at the end of the bed.
- Keep the patient in good alignment, in the center of the bed.
- Make sure that the body is acting properly as countertraction by keeping the head of the bed low.
- The feet should not rest against the end of the bed.
- Check under halters or straps for areas of pressure or irritation.
- Make sure straps of halters and belts are smooth, straight, and properly secured.
- Keep bed covers off ropes and pulleys.

Fractured Hip

Hip fractures are the most common type of fracture in the elderly. The most common cause of hip fractures is falls, but they occasionally occur because of osteoporosis.

Signs and Symptoms of Hip Fracture

A patient with a fractured hip is usually found on the floor. He or she will be unable to get up or to move the injured leg. The leg on the affected side may be shortened and in a position of external rotation. In this position, the toes point outward. The shortening and rotation occur because the strong muscles in the upper leg contract, causing the bone ends to override each other. The patient will complain of severe pain in the hip.

The pain of a hip fracture is usually localized in the hip. Some patients complain of pain in the knee, which may be confusing or misleading. Edema and ecchymosis may be present in the hip, thigh, groin, or lower pelvic area.

Emergency Care

Avoid moving the patient until you are instructed to do so by a nurse. You will use a sheet, backboard, or other device to move the patient. Avoid excessive movement, which can worsen the injury. Moving a patient with a hip fracture requires four or five individuals. The patient is logrolled onto the lifting device, and the device is then lifted to the bed or stretcher. You may be assigned to monitor the patient's vital signs and check for signs of shock.

Open Reduction/Internal Fixation

The most common treatment for a fractured hip is a surgical procedure called open reduction/internal fixation. If you are assigned to a patient who has had this surgery, you must:
- Know how to position the patient in bed. It is important to avoid adduction and internal and external rotation of the affected hip.
- Know the correct procedure if the patient is allowed to ambulate. The patient must not be allowed to bear weight on the affected side for a few weeks after surgery.

Total Hip Arthroplasty

Total hip arthroplasty (THA), or insertion of a hip prosthesis (artificial body part), is a common procedure.

Guidelines for Caring for Patients with Total Hip Arthroplasty

The patient should **not**:
- Flex the hip more than 90 degrees (Figure 11-3A).

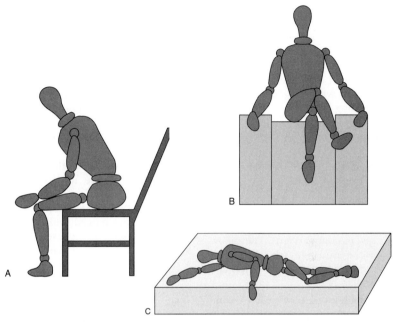

Figure 11-3 A patient with a new hip prosthesis should never: (A) flex the affected hip more than 90 degrees. (B) cross the affected leg over the midline of the body. (C) externally rotate the affected hip.

- Cross the affected leg over the midline of the body, whether in bed or sitting in a chair (Figure 11-3B).
- Internally rotate the hip on the affected side (Figure 11-3C).

Never do passive range-of-motion exercises on a joint that has had surgery, unless you are specifically instructed to do so—and then only if you have been given instructions as to which actions can safely be performed.

The patient will have limited weight bearing on the affected leg for several days or weeks after surgery.

Caring for the Patient with Hip Surgery

After hip surgery, the following general procedures are commonly ordered:

- A trapeze is attached to the bed to assist with movement. The patient is instructed not to press down on the foot of the affected leg when using the trapeze.
- Antiembolism stockings are applied.
- A fracture bedpan is used initially for elimination. When the patient is able to use the toilet, an elevated toilet seat is used.
- The head of the bed is not elevated more than 45 degrees without a specific order.
- Avoid acute flexion of the hip and legs. The physician will give directions for positioning and the degree of flexion permitted.
- Patients who have had hip replacement surgery will usually have a special pillow, called an abduction pillow, to keep the legs apart. This is particularly important when the patient is turned on the side. The patient will be instructed to avoid crossing the legs, which can cause a dislocation.

Nursing Assistant Role

- Assist with procedures to prevent the complications of immobility.
- Provide range-of-motion exercises of the unaffected extremities.
- Assist with turning and repositioning, and with coughing and deep breathing exercises.
- Prevent skin breakdown, especially on the heels. Relieve pressure from the heels and check the patient's skin carefully each day for signs of red or open areas.
- The care plan will specify when to use the abduction pillow. This is important in patients with THA to prevent complications. The pillow may be used in both bed and chair, according to physicians' orders and the plan of care.
- Antiembolism hosiery are commonly used for patients with hip surgery to prevent blood clots. Make sure the hosiery are the correct size. The hosiery must be smooth and wrinkle free so they do not interfere with circulation or increase pressure. Check the hole in the toe end as specified on the care plan to monitor circulation. Remove the hosiery regularly for bathing and as ordered. Monitor the skin daily for signs of redness or breakdown. If the patient complains of pain in the foot or toes, remove the hosiery so the area can be visualized. Inform the nurse so he or she can assess the circulation before the hosiery are reapplied.

Total Joint Replacement

Various joints can be completely replaced because of arthritis or severe damage to the joint. The goal of joint replacement surgery is to relieve pain, which is often so severe that the patient avoids using the joint as much as possible. General care for joint replacement surgery includes:

- Preventing infection
- Preventing blood clots
- Administering anticoagulant medication to thin the blood
- Applying antiembolism hosiery
- Exercises to increase blood flow in the leg muscles, if not contraindicated
- Sequential compression therapy

Continuous Passive Motion

Continuous passive motion (CPM) therapy prevents stiffness by delivering a form of passive range of motion so the joint is moved without the patient's muscles being used. CPM therapy is effortless for the patient. A machine moves the affected joint through a prescribed range of motion for an extended period of time.

The physician prescribes how the CPM unit should be used. The directions for use will vary slightly depending on the body area being treated, the type of CPM machine used, and physicians' orders. In some facilities, this procedure is done only by licensed nurses. In others, the nursing assistant can set up the unit, but the nurse must check the settings for accuracy.

This is a key step. Improper settings can damage reconstructive work in the joint. Follow your facility policies and procedures.

Contraindications for CPM therapy:

- Untreated infections
- Unstable fractures
- Known or suspected blood clots (deep vein thrombosis)
- Hemorrhage

If the patient develops any of the following signs or symptoms upon using the device, stop the unit and inform the nurse promptly:

- Fever
- Increasing redness or irritation

- Increasing warmth
- Edema
- Bleeding
- Increased or persistent pain

Do not proceed with treatment until the nurse informs you that the physician has approved continued use of the device.

- Check the patient periodically when using the CPM machine.
- Each time the settings are changed, stay with the patient for several cycles to be sure he or she tolerates the change.
- Check the skin every 2 hours for signs of redness, irritation, or breakdown.
- Report problems and abnormalities to the nurse.

Compartment Syndrome

Compartment syndrome is a very painful condition that occurs when pressure within the muscles builds up, preventing blood and oxygen from reaching muscles and nerves. Compartment syndrome is usually seen after a traumatic injury, such as a fracture of a long bone. It may develop if an injury or surgical site swells after a cast has been applied. If blood flow is not restored promptly, tissue death begins.

Signs and Symptoms

The most common symptom of acute compartment syndrome is severe pain, especially when the muscle is moved. The pain may seem out of proportion to the injury. The patient may also complain of

- Severe pain when the muscle is stretched gently
- Tenderness when the area is touched gently
- Pain on deep breathing in some patients
- Tingling

- Burning
- Numbness
- Feeling tight or full in the affected muscle
- Abnormal sensations in the affected area
- Weakness or inability to use the muscle

You may observe:

- The color of the extremity may appear pale, cyanotic, or red.
- The skin of an extremity with no cast may feel warm to the touch.
- The fingers or toes of a casted extremity may feel cool to the touch.
- Edema (swelling).

Loss of the pulse in the extremity is a late sign. Rapid identification and treatment of this condition is necessary.

The most common location of compartment syndrome in adults is in a fractured tibia. The most common location of compartment syndrome in children is the humerus.

Nursing Assistant Responsibilities

- Follow the care plan.
- Monitor patients with musculoskeletal injuries and casts frequently.
- Monitor for changes in the extremity.
- Check the color and temperature of the extremity distal to a cast.
- Ask the patient if he or she is able to move fingers or toes.
- Notify the nurse promptly of any unusual findings.
- If the patient complains of severe pain, or if the pain is not relieved after the patient receives pain medication, notify the nurse promptly.
- Provide emotional support.

If compartment syndrome is suspected, the patient will be taken to surgery quickly to relieve the pressure. Follow facility policies and the nurse's instructions for preparing the patient for surgery.

Lower Extremity Amputation

You may care for patients who have had one or both legs amputated. It is common for people to experience phantom pain after the removal of a limb. Patients with phantom pain may feel pain or tingling where the limb used to be. These feelings may persist for months. The pain is caused by severing and altering the nerves during surgery. It is real, not imaginary, and can be quite severe. Inform the nurse promptly if the patient complains of pain.

When you are positioning a patient who has had an amputation of the lower extremities, remember:

- Avoid abduction and flexion of the patient's hip—because the weight of the lower leg is not there, the hip on the affected side will quickly become contracted if flexion is allowed.
- If the patient has a below-the-knee amputation (BKA), avoid flexion of the knee so that a contracture does not form.
- Avoid placing pillows under the amputated extremity. Position the leg flat on the bed.
- Avoid elevating the head of the bed for prolonged periods of time.
- Keep the legs in a position of adduction. A trochanter roll is helpful. Avoid positioning the patient with pillows between the legs.
- Assist the patient to lie in the prone position twice a day, if permitted.
- Encourage and assist the patient to move in bed frequently.
- After the surgery, the patient either will have the stump wrapped with elastic bandage or will wear a garment to shape the stump, called a stump shrinker. It is important that these be on at all times except during bathing.
- If you notice that the bandage or shrinker is loose or needs to be reapplied, notify the nurse.
- Inform the nurse promptly if the patient complains of throbbing under the stump shrinker. Throbbing is an indication of impaired circulation, a potentially serious complication.

If you bathe a patient with an amputation:

- Gently wash the stump with soap and warm water, rinse well, and pat dry.
- Observe the stump for:
  - Redness
  - Swelling
  - Drainage from the incision
  - Open areas in the incision or anywhere else on the stump
- Do not apply lotion or powder to the stump. Lotion softens the skin, making safe prosthesis use difficult.
- Make sure the skin is protected before applying the prosthesis. Never apply a prosthesis over unprotected skin.
- If you are responsible for helping a patient put on a prosthesis, be sure you know how to attach and secure it.
- Avoid shaving the stump; shaving increases the risk of rash and irritation.
- Bathing the stump may be ordered at bedtime because warm water may increase swelling, making application of the prosthesis difficult.
- The physician may also order alcohol rubs to the stump several times a day to toughen the skin.
- Monitor the stump for irritation and report to the nurse, if present.
- The stump socks may require frequent changing to avoid wetness.

The socks must be washed by hand.

- Muscle-strengthening exercises will be ordered to prepare the patient to lift the weight of the prosthesis.

RANGE OF MOTION

Patients' joints must be moved regularly to prevent complications.

- Active range-of-motion (AROM) exercises are done by the patient during activities of daily living.
- Passive range-of-motion (PROM) exercises are performed for patients when independent movement is impossible.

AROM maintains movement, prevents deformity, and strengthens muscles. PROM exercises are performed for patients when independent movement is impossible, such as when the patient has existing contractures or paralysis. PROM exercises maintain movement and prevent deformities, but do not strengthen the muscles. Exercises also stimulate circulation and improve body function.

You may also see orders for two other types of range of motion on the care plan. Active and passive range of motion are routinely done on many types of nursing units. The other two types are more commonly done in therapy, as part of a restorative nursing program, or in a rehabilitation unit or subacute center. These are:

- *Active assistive range of motion (AAROM)* exercises may also be called *active assisted range of motion*. These exercises are either started or completed by the patient. The exercises are done when the patient needs assistance moving because of paralysis, weakness or paresis, pain, or spasticity. However, the assistance is limited to only what is needed by the patient. Practice and profiency are needed

so you know how much hands-on assistance is right for each patient. Occasionally, verbal cues and demonstration are the only measures needed. Occasionally, equipment, such as elastic straps, pulleys, or rubber balls, are used for exercising joints. This is another form of active assistive range of motion.

- *Resistive range of motion (RROM)* exercises are ordered to increase strength. Patients work against manual or mechanical resistance. At the beginning of the exercise program, the resistance is slight. The amount of resistance is increased as the patient develops strength and endurance.

If the care plan lists AAROM or RROM exercises, be sure you have been taught to perform these activities and are permitted to do them in your facility. If you have questions or concerns, discuss them with the nurse.

The patient must be comfortable and relaxed during the exercises. Each joint is taken through the normal range of movement.

The nurse will instruct you as to the type or limitation of range-of-motion exercises to be done. These exercises are usually done during or after the bath and before the bed is made.

Guidelines for Assisting Patients with Range-of-Motion Exercises

- Check the care plan or with the nurse for specific guidelines and limitations.
- Explain the procedure to the patient.
- Before beginning, make sure the patient is comfortable.
- Position the patient in good body alignment, in the supine position, before beginning.

- Elevate the bed to a comfortable working height.
- Use good posture and apply the principles of good body mechanics.
- Encourage the patient to assist, if able, but keep your hands in position to provide support.
- Make sure you have enough space for full movement of the extremities.
- Expose only the part of the body you are exercising.
- Support each joint by placing one hand above and one hand below the joint.
- Move each joint slowly and consistently. Stop briefly at the end of each motion.
- Work systematically from top of the body to bottom.
- Never push the patient past the point of joint resistance. Move each joint as far as it will comfortably go.
- In many facilities, the neck is not exercised without a physician's order. Know and follow your facility policy.
- Perform each joint motion five times, or according to facility policy.
- Stop the exercise and report to the nurse if the patient complains of pain. Watch the patient's body language and facial expression for signs of pain.
- Be alert for changes in the patient's condition during the activity. If you feel that the activity is harming the patient, stop. Notify a nurse. Changes that suggest a potential problem are pain, shortness of breath, sweating, and change in color.
- Help the patient relax during exercise.
- Use this time to communicate with the patient.
- For patients who are stiff or combative, consider doing the exercise

in the bathtub or whirlpool. Check with the nurse.

PROCEDURE: PERFORMING RANGE-OF-MOTION EXERCISES (PASSIVE)

Note: This procedure may be carried out as an independent procedure or as part of the bath. Repeat each action five times. ROM is described here as an independent procedure.

Caution: Passive range of motion that involves the neck is usually carried out by a physical therapist or a registered nurse. Patients who can exercise this area themselves are encouraged to do so. Check your facility policy regarding ROM neck exercises.

1. Carry out each beginning procedure action.
2. Assemble equipment: bath blanket.
3. Position patient on back close to you.
4. Adjust the bath blanket to keep patient covered as much as possible.
5. Supporting the elbow and wrist, exercise shoulder joint nearest you as follows:
   a. Bring the entire arm out at right angle to the body (horizontal abduction) (Figure 11-4).
   b. Return the arm to a position parallel to the body (horizontal adduction).
6. a. With arm parallel to the body, roll entire arm toward body (internal rotation of shoulder).
   b. Maintaining the parallel position, roll entire arm away from body (external rotation of shoulder).
7. With shoulder in abduction, flex elbow and raise entire arm overhead (shoulder flexion) (Figure 11-5).

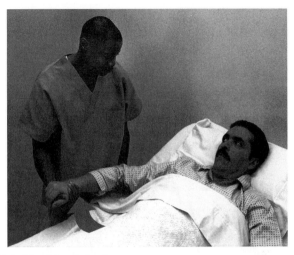

Figure 11-4 Shoulder abduction.

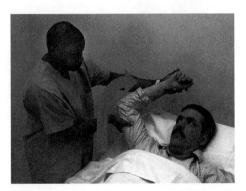

Figure 11-5 Shoulder flexion.

8. With arm parallel to body (palm up—supination), flex and extend elbow (Figures 11-6A, B).

9. Flex and extend wrist (Figure 11-7A). Flex and extend each finger joint (Figure 11-7B).

10. Move each finger, in turn, away from the middle finger (abduction) (Figure 11-8A) and toward the middle finger (adduction) (Figure 11-8B).

11. Abduct the thumb by moving it toward the extended fingers (Figure 11-9A).

12. Touch the thumb to the base of the little finger, then to each fingertip (opposition) (Figure 11-9B).

13. Turn hand palm down (pronation), then palm up (supination).

14. Grasp patient's wrist with one hand and patient's hand with the other. Bring wrist toward body (inversion) and then away from the body (eversion) (Figure 11-10).

15. Point hand in supination toward thumb side (radial deviation), then toward little-finger side (ulnar deviation).

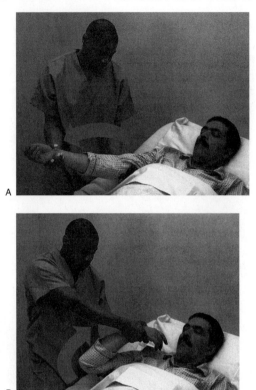

A

B

Figure 11-6 (A) Elbow extension; (B) elbow flexion.

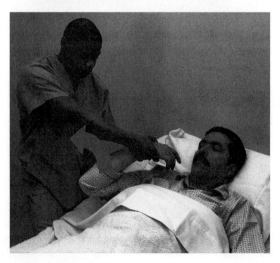

Figure 11-7A Wrist extension.

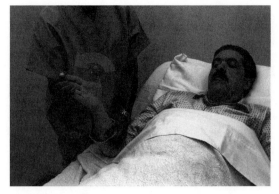

Figure 11-7B Finger extension.

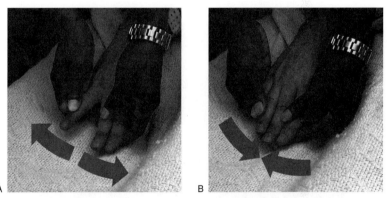

A   B

Figure 11-8 (A) Finger abduction; (B) finger adduction.

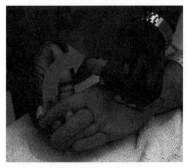

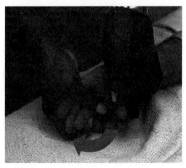

Figure 11-9A Thumb adduction.   **Figure 11-9B** Thumb opposition.

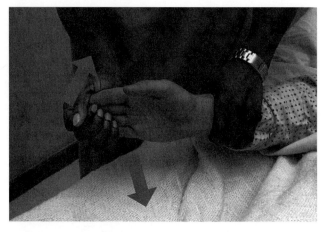

Figure 11-10 Wrist inversion (supination) and eversion (pronation).

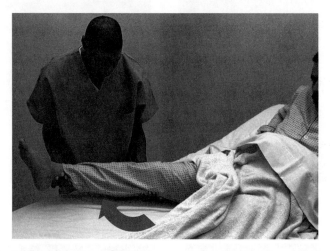

Figure 11-11 Abduction of the hip.

16. Cover patient's upper extremities and body. Expose only the leg being exercised. Face the foot of the bed.

17. Supporting the knee and ankle, move the entire leg away from body center (abduction) (Figure 11-11) and toward the body (adduction).

18. Turn to face bed. Supporting the knee in bent position (flexion), raise the knee toward the pelvis (hip flexion) (Figure 11-12). Straighten the knee (extension) as you lower the leg to the bed.

19. a. Supporting the leg at knee and ankle, roll the leg in a circular fashion away from the body (lateral hip rotation).

    b. Continuing to support leg, roll leg in the same fashion toward the body (medial hip rotation).

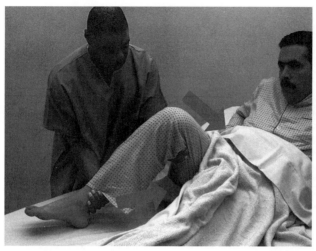

Figure 11-12 Hip and knee flexion.

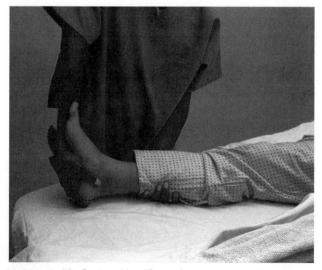

Figure 11-13A Ankle flexion (dorsiflexion).

20. Grasp patient's toes and support ankle. Bring toes toward the knee (dorsiflexion) (Figure 11-13A). Then point toes toward the foot of the bed (plantar flexion) (Figure 11-13B).

Note: *The patient may be more comfortable if the knee is slightly flexed during this motion.*

21. Gently turn patient's foot inward (inversion) and outward (eversion).

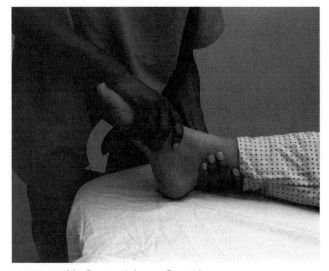

Figure 11-13B Ankle flexion (plantar flexion).

22. Place your fingers over patient's toes. Bend toes (flexion) and straighten toes (extension).

23. Move each toe away from the second toe (abduction) (Figure 11-14A) and then toward the second toe (adduction) (Figure 11-14B).

24. Cover the leg with the bath blanket. Raise the side rail and move to the opposite side of the bed.

25. Move the patient close to you and repeat steps 5 through 24.

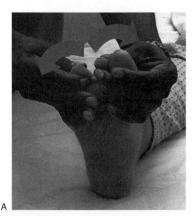
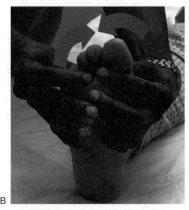

A   B

Figure 11-14 (A) Toe abduction; (B) toe adduction.

DISORDERS OF THE ENDOCRINE SYSTEM

The endocrine glands are subject to disease that can result in hyposecretion (underproduction) and hypersecretion (overproduction) of hormones. Hormones are chemicals that regulate the body's activities.

COMMON CONDITIONS OF THE THYROID GLAND

The thyroid gland may secrete too much or not enough hormones. Either situation is treatable. If not treated, severe illness or death will occur.

Hyperthyroidism

Hyperthyroidism, or overactivity of the thyroid gland, results in production of too much thyroxine (hypersecretion). The person shows:
- Irritability and restlessness
- Nervousness
- Rapid pulse
- Increased appetite
- Weight loss
- Sensitivity

Nursing Assistant Actions
- Be understanding and have patience.
- Keep the room quiet and cool.
- Encourage good nutrition.

Thyroidectomy
It may be necessary to treat hyperthyroidism with surgery. You may be assigned to assist in the postoperative care. Following surgery:
- The patient is placed in a semi-Fowler's position, with neck and shoulders well supported. Remember at all times to support the back of the neck. Hyperextension of the neck may damage the operative site.
- Assist with oxygen, if ordered, using all oxygen precautions.
- Give routine postoperative care.
- Check for and report the following:
  - Any signs of bleeding (this may drain toward the back of the neck). Check the pillows behind the patient, as well as the dressings.
  - Signs of respiratory distress.
  - Inability of the patient to speak. Initial hoarseness is common, but any increase should be reported.
  - Greatly elevated temperature and pulse, pronounced apprehension, or irritability.
  - Numbness, tingling, or muscular spasm (tetany) of the extremities.

DIABETES MELLITUS

Diabetes mellitus is a chronic disease that results from a deficiency of insulin or a resistance to the effects of insulin. Glucose from the breakdown of food remains in the blood, resulting in elevated blood sugar. Persistent, elevated glucose levels affect the blood vessels and nerves, making the person with diabetes more likely to develop heart attack, stroke, blindness, renal disease, and other serious complications and conditions.

The incidence of diabetes mellitus increases as people age.

Types of Diabetes Mellitus

Diabetes mellitus is typed and named according to the need for insulin. Examples are:

- Insulin-dependent diabetes mellitus (IDDM), which has an onset in childhood
- Non-insulin-dependent diabetes (NIDDM), which is more common in adults, but is increasingly seen in children.

Care of the diabetic is directed toward maintaining a normal blood glucose level so that complications may be prevented. To regulate blood glucose, the diabetic person must:

- Eat a healthful, well-balanced diet as prescribed by the physician.
- Exercise regularly in a manner appropriate for the person's age and ability.
- Check the blood sugar regularly.
- Use insulin or oral antidiabetic agents correctly if ordered by the physician.
- Control weight.

Hypoglycemic Drugs

Diabetes mellitus is treated by one of two main drug groups. One is administered subcutaneously or through a tiny pump. The other is given orally. *Note: When insulin is self-administered, it is important to report any missed injections or signs of infection around the administration site.*

Hypoglycemia (Low Blood Sugar)

Hypoglycemia occurs when the blood glucose level is below normal. It:

- May occur rapidly
- Is referred to as insulin reaction or

insulin shock when caused by an overdose of insulin

Hypoglycemia can be brought on by:

- Skipping meals
- Unusual activity
- Stress
- Vomiting
- Diarrhea
- Omission of planned snack or meals
- Interaction of drugs
- Too much insulin or oral hypoglycemic medications

Signs and Symptoms

The signs and symptoms of hypoglycemia include:

- Complaints of hunger, weakness, dizziness, shakiness
- Skin cold, moist, clammy, pale
- Rapid, shallow respirations
- Nervousness and excitement
- Rapid pulse
- Unconsciousness
- No sugar in the urine
- Low blood sugar by finger stick

If the patient is awake and alert, treatment includes intake of orange juice, milk, or another easily absorbed carbohydrate such as hard candy.

Hyperglycemia (High Blood Sugar)

Hyperglycemia (diabetic coma)

- Occurs when there is insufficient insulin for metabolic needs
- Usually develops slowly, sometimes over a 24-hour period
- May be seen as confusion, drowsiness, or a slow slippage into coma in a patient who is confined to bed

Hyperglycemia may be brought on by:

- Stress
- Illness such as infection
- Dehydration
- Injury

- Forgotten medication
- Intake of too much food

Signs and Symptoms

The signs and symptoms of diabetic coma include:

- Early headache, drowsiness, or confusion
- Sweet, fruity odor to the breath
- Deep breathing
- Labored respirations
- Full, bounding pulse
- Low blood pressure
- Nausea or vomiting
- Flushed, dry, hot skin
- Weakness
- Unconsciousness
- Sugar in the urine
- High blood sugar by finger stick

Nursing Assistant Responsibilities

- Know the signs of insulin shock and diabetic coma.
- Be alert for the signs of diabetic coma or insulin shock and report them immediately to the nurse.
- Know the storage location of orange juice or other easily absorbed sources of carbohydrates.
- Keep easily absorbed carbohydrates, such as orange juice, crackers, or hard candy, available if caring for the diabetic patient at home.
- Check the food tray to ensure the food is allowed on the patient's diet.
- Do not give extra nourishment without permission.
- Keep a record of the patient's food consumption.
- Report uneaten meals to the nurse.
- Give special attention to care of the diabetic patient's feet.
  - Wash daily, carefully drying between the toes.
  - Inspect feet closely for any breaks or signs of irritation.
  - Report any abnormalities to the nurse.
  - Keep the area between the toes dry.
  - The toenails of a diabetic should be cut only by a podiatrist, a doctor who specializes in foot care.
- Shoes and stockings should be clean, free of holes, and fit well. Anything that might injure the feet or interfere with the circulation must be avoided.
- Do not allow the patient to go barefoot or wear shoes without socks.
- Report signs and symptoms of infection, even if they seem minor.

Blood Glucose Monitoring

Bedside glucose testing has become very common in the management of patients with diabetes. Many individuals perform this testing at home several times each day. The antidiabetic medication may be adjusted according to the patient's blood sugar. A blood sample is taken from a capillary. The test meter will display the blood sugar value in 1 minute or less. Nursing assistants perform this procedure in some facilities. Know and follow your facility policy. If you are responsible for this procedure, you should:

- Collect the capillary sample exactly as ordered. Specimens that are not collected at the proper time can cause misinterpretation of the results.
- Always report the value to the nurse.
- Document according to facility policy.
- If the nurse asks you to obtain a stat blood sugar, do so immediately.
- Report the results immediately.

Fingerstick Blood Sugar

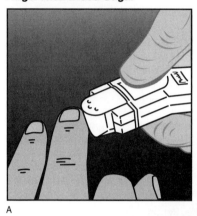 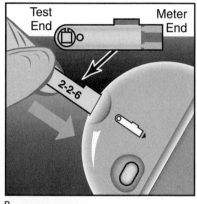

A   B

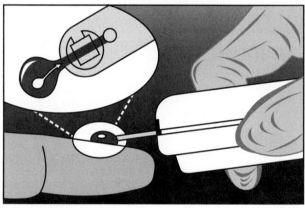

C

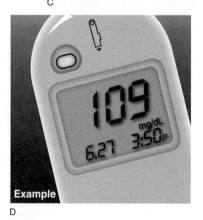

D

Fingerstick blood sugar (FSBS) is checked by collecting a sample of capillary blood with a lancet, or tiny needle (Figure 12-1A–D). The blood is transferred to a reagent strip or other test strip. For most reagent strips, you must place a hanging drop of blood onto the reagent pad. Avoid smearing the strip against the finger. Most newer meters have a tiny tube that draws blood to the inside on contact. An audible beep informs you when the tube has collected enough blood.

Figure 12-1 Using a glucometer: (A) Pierce the side of the finger with the lancet. (B) Insert the strip in the meter. (C) The strip draws blood into the meter. (D) Read the meter after the designated period of time.

Many different blood glucose meters are available. Each meter has its own reagent or test strip. For accuracy:

- Make sure the strip is compatible with the meter you are using.
- Do not use the strips beyond the expiration date.
- Follow the directions for the meter and reagent strips you are using.
- Discard lancets into the puncture-resistant sharps container.
- Avoid cross-contamination of equipment.

The normal blood sugar values vary with the health care facility. The normal fasting range in most facilities is somewhere between 65 mg/dl and 120 mg/dl, with the normal value commonly being 70 mg/dl to 110 mg/dl. Values below 70 mg/dl always suggest hypoglycemia. Fasting values above 110 mg/dl suggest hyperglycemia.

Notify the nurse immediately of blood sugar values outside of the normal range or of other signs and symptoms of blood sugar problems, such as:

- Inadequate food intake
- Eating food not permitted on diet
- Refusal of meals, supplements, or snacks
- Nausea, vomiting, or diarrhea
- Inadequate fluid intake
- Excessive activity
- Complaints of dizziness, shakiness, racing heart

Some blood glucose meters do not have a wide range. If the screen displays the word "low" or "high," the patient has the potential for serious complications. His or her condition may deteriorate quickly. Inform the nurse immediately.

Acetone Monitoring

Ketone bodies are created when body fat is burned as an alternative source of fuel to sugar. The ketone bodies incite a chemical imbalance, causing acids to accumulate and upsetting the patient's buffer system. If a patient's blood sugar is over 250 mg/dl, the nurse may instruct you to check the patient's urine for ketones. If the patient is very ill, the nurse may request a ketone test even if the blood sugar is not high.

GLYCATED HEMOGLOBIN

Glycated hemoglobin is a term used to describe a series of stable minor hemoglobin components formed from hemoglobin and glucose. It is commonly called "A1c," which is the abbreviation we will use here. This test measures blood glucose levels for a 3-month period. It is very useful to the doctor because he or she can tell if the patient's diabetes is under good control at home.

The American Diabetes Association (ADA) recommends hemoglobin A1c testing twice a year for patients who are meeting treatment goals, and four times a year for patients who are not meeting their goals, as well as those who need more intensive monitoring. Home testing kits are now available. The single use, disposable kits are also being used in physicians' offices, and as a point of care bedside test in the hospital and long term care facility.

Patient teaching is a very important part of patient care for patients with diabetes. Being able to evaluate the patient's diabetic control at home also enables the RN and certified diabetes educator to plan and provide patient teaching. The information helps the dietitian to assist the patient with diet management, food preparation, and methods of meeting the patient's individual dietary wants and needs. A conversion chart of A1c values is listed in Table 12-1.

Table 12-1   CONVERSION CHART GLYCATED HEMOGLOBIN A1c AND BLOOD GLUCOSE

HEMOGLOBIN A1c	APPROXIMATE AVERAGE DAILY BLOOD GLUCOSE
12.0%	345 mg/dl
11.0%	310 mg/dl
10.0%	275 mg/dl
9.0%	240 mg/dl
8.0%	205 mg/dl
7.0%	170 mg/dl
6.0%	135 mg/dl
5.0%	100 mg/dl
4.0%	65 mg/dl

DISORDERS OF THE NERVOUS SYSTEM

The nervous system usually remains healthy. However, injury or disease involving the brain, spinal cord, or nerves requires appropriate treatment.

INCREASED INTRACRANIAL PRESSURE

The structures within the skull normally exert a certain amount of pressure, called the intracranial pressure. The pressure is due to:

- Nervous tissue
- Cerebrospinal fluid
- Blood flowing through the cerebral vessels

Any change in the size or amount of these components changes the pressure.

Signs and Symptoms

Indications of increased intracranial pressure include:

- Alteration in pupil size and response to light. In the normal eye, the pupil becomes smaller when a flashlight is directed at each eye. The equality of the pupils and their ability to react to light are important observations when a head injury occurs.
- Headache.
- Vomiting.
- Loss of consciousness and sensation.
- Paralysis—loss of voluntary motor control.

- Convulsions (seizures)—uncontrolled muscular contractions that are often violent.

How long all or part of the symptoms remain depends on the extent and cause of damage to the brain cells. Remember also that paralysis is not always accompanied by sensory loss.

Specific Nursing Care

Patients who are acutely ill with head injuries or increased intracranial pressure require skilled nursing care. If you note any change in the patient's response or behavior as you are assisting in care, bring it to the nurse's attention immediately. Changes that might be very significant include new onset:

- Incontinence
- Uncontrolled body movements
- Disorientation
- Deepening or lessening in the level of consciousness
- Dizziness
- Vomiting
- Alterations in speech
- Change in ability to follow directions

Loss of sensation and decreased mobility make these patients more prone to pressure ulcers, infection, and contractures. You must continue to:

- Give special skin care.
- Carry out range-of-motion exercises.
- Check skin over pressure points frequently.

111

- Change the patient's position regularly.
- Report early signs of infection.
- Monitor elimination. Loss of muscle tone and inactivity may lead to constipation and impaction.
- Check drainage tubes such as indwelling catheters. They must receive careful attention.
- Provide reality orientation as needed.
- Be alert to any signs of mood changes and plan extra time to provide emotional support.
- Keep a careful check on vital signs for any patient with a head injury. A special neurological monitoring record may be kept for all observations.
- The Glasgow Coma Scale is used to monitor neurological problems after trauma, stroke, and other illnesses and injuries. Higher point values are assigned to responses that indicate increased awareness and arousal. A score of less than 8 indicates a neurological crisis. A score of 9 to 13 indicates moderate dysfunction, and a score of 13 to 15 indicates moderate to minor dysfunction.

STROKE

A stroke is also called a cerebrovascular accident (CVA) or brain attack. It affects the vascular system and the nervous system. The complete or partial loss of blood flow to the brain tissue is frequently a complication of atherosclerosis or brain hemorrhage. Causes of CVA include:

- Vascular occlusion due to a thrombus, atherosclerotic plaques, or emboli that obstruct the flow of blood
- Intracranial bleeding as blood vessels rupture, releasing blood into the brain tissue

Remember, most nerve pathways cross. Therefore, damage on one side of the brain results in signs and symptoms on the opposite side of the body. Symptoms vary depending on the extent of interference with the circulation and on the area and amount of tissue damaged. Patients with damage to the right side of the brain may exhibit:

- Paralysis on the left side of the body (left hemiplegia).
- Spatial-perceptual deficits, in which the patient has difficulty distinguishing right from left and up from down.
- Change in personality. The individual with right brain damage becomes very quick and impulsive.

If the left side of the brain is damaged, you may note:
- Paralysis on the right side of the body (right hemiplegia).
- Aphasia—an inability to express or understand speech.
- Change in personality. The individual becomes very cautious, anxious, and slow to complete tasks.

Other symptoms may be present with either right-brain or left-brain damage. These include:
- Sensory-perceptual deficits
  - Loss of position sense. The person cannot tell, for example, where an affected foot is or what position it is in without looking at it.
  - The inability to identify common objects such as a comb, a fork, a pencil, or a glass.
  - The inability to use common objects.
- Unilateral neglect. The patient ignores the paralyzed side of the body.

- Hemianopsia. This is impaired vision. Both eyes have only half vision. If the patient has left hemiplegia, the left half of both eyes is blind. Remember this if a patient who has had a stroke eats the food on one side of the tray and leaves the food on the other side. The patient probably cannot see it. Turn the tray around.
- Emotional liability. Patients who have had a stroke may start to cry or laugh for no apparent reason. They have very little control over this and may be embarrassed.
- Cognitive impairments. There may be changes in the patient's intellectual function. This may affect memory, judgment, and problem-solving abilities.

Nursing Care

The goals of poststroke care include:
- Maintaining the skills and abilities that the patient has left
- Preventing complications caused by immobility:
  – Contractures
  – Pressure ulcers
  – Pneumonia
  – Blood clots

- Helping the patient regain functional abilities:
  – Activities of daily living
  – Bowel and bladder control
  – Mobility
  – Communication skills

Communicating with a Patient Who Has Had a CVA

- Find the most effective means of communicating the information you need to convey.
- Ask yes or no questions whenever possible.
- Avoid treating the patient like a child, and do not correct his or her speech.
- If you must repeat yourself, do so quietly and calmly.
- Use gestures, if necessary.

APHASIA

Stroke victims often suffer from aphasia, or language impairment. They have difficulty forming thoughts or expressing them in coherent ways. This is extremely frustrating and frightening to the patient and family.

- Receptive aphasia means that the person cannot comprehend communication.
- Expressive aphasia means that the person cannot properly form thoughts or express them coherently.
- Global aphasia means that the person has lost all language abilities.

PARKINSON'S DISEASE

Parkinson's disease is believed to be caused by not having enough neurotransmitters (dopamine) in the brain stem and cerebellum. The symptoms are progressive over many years. Some people will show minor changes. Others will have much more obvious symptoms.

Signs and Symptoms

Signs and symptoms of Parkinson's disease include:
- Tremors (uncontrolled trembling).
- Muscular rigidity (loss of flexibility), which is more evident when the person is inactive.
- Akinesia (difficulty and slowness in carrying out voluntary muscular activities). Persons with advanced Parkinson's typically have:
  – A shuffling manner of walking
  – Difficulty starting the process of walking

- Difficulty stopping smoothly once walking has started
- Affected speech, causing words to be slurred and poorly spoken (enunciated)
- Facial muscles that lose expressiveness and emotional response
• Loss of autonomic nervous control, which may cause:
  - Drooling
  - Incontinence
  - Constipation
  - Urinary retention
• Mood swings and gradual behavioral changes.
• Depression.
• Dementia in later stages.

Nursing Assistant Care

Nursing care of the person with Parkinson's disease includes:
• Maintaining a calm, stress-free environment. Symptoms are more intense when the patient is under stress.
• Assisting and supervising the activities of daily living.
• Providing emotional support and encouragement.
• Carrying out a program of general and specific exercises.
• Supervising or assisting with ambulation and mobility.
• Providing protection for patients with dementia.

MULTIPLE SCLEROSIS

Multiple sclerosis (MS) generally occurs in young adults. It is the result of the loss of insulation (myelin) around central nervous system nerve fibers. This interferes with the ability of the nerve fibers to function. Symptoms may include:
• Loss of sensation with regard to temperature, pain, and touch

• Feelings of numbness and tingling
• Vertigo (a spinning or dizzy sensation)
• Lhermitte's sign (a tingling, shock-like sensation that passes down the arms or spine when the neck is flexed)
• Blurriness, color blindness, or difficulty seeing objects in bright light
• Double vision
• Nystagmus (jerky eye movements)

Mobility is usually affected:
• Pain in the legs that disappears with rest
• Paraplegia (paralysis of both legs) and tetraplegia (paralysis of all four extremities) in advanced cases
• Spasticity of muscles
• Intention tremor (shaking of the hands that gets worse as the individual tries to touch or pick up an object)
• In severe MS, speech is affected because of the weakness of the muscles in the chest, face, and lips. The speech may be slow, with poor articulation. The mind usually remains alert. Incontinence of the bowel and bladder are common in advanced cases. One of the most disabling features of MS is fatigue.

Nursing Assistant Care

Nursing care of the patient with multiple sclerosis includes:
• Implement pressure ulcer prevention program.
• Implement contracture prevention programs through consistent changes of position and passive range-of-motion exercises. Apply splints correctly, if ordered.
• Pay careful attention to catheter care if the patient has an indwelling catheter, to prevent bladder infections.

- Encourage independence. Follow instructions of nurse or the therapists for specific techniques to use.
- Help the patient maintain a balanced schedule of rest and activity.
- Provide emotional support and encouragement.

SEIZURE DISORDER (EPILEPSY)

Seizure disorder (convulsions, epilepsy) involves recurrent, transient attacks of disturbed brain function. It is characterized by various forms of convulsions called seizures. Not all seizures are alike.

There are many different types and categories of seizure activity. The most common types of seizure activity are classified as follows:

- Partial seizures
  - There may or may not be a loss of consciousness.
  - Seizures generally begin in one part of the body and involve only one side of the body.
- Generalized seizures
  - These include grand mal seizures and are also known as generalized tonic-clonic seizures. There is bilateral generalized motor movement and muscular rigidity. Consciousness is lost, and an aura may occur in the form of lights, sounds, or aromas at the beginning of the seizure. When this seizure begins, the patient cries out, then falls to the floor. The muscles stiffen (tonic phase), then the extremities begin to jerk and twitch (clonic phase). The patient may lose bladder control. Consciousness returns slowly. After this seizure, the patient may feel tired or be

confused and disoriented. This may last from a few minutes to several hours or days. The patient may fall asleep or gradually become less confused until full consciousness returns.
  - Petit mal seizures are characterized by momentary loss of muscle tone. These are also called absence seizures. The seizure begins without warning and consists of a period of unconsciousness, in which the patient blinks rapidly, stares blankly, breathes rapidly, or makes chewing movements. The seizure lasts 2 to 10 seconds, then ends abruptly. The patient usually resumes normal activity immediately.
- Status epilepticus is a seizure that lasts for a long time or that repeats without recovery. It is a serious medical emergency. Death may result if the patient is not treated immediately. Status epilepticus can be convulsive (tonic-clonic) or nonconvulsive (absence).

Nursing Assistant Care During Seizures

The main nursing focus during a seizure is to:

- Prevent injury by:
  - Staying with the person
  - Assisting the person to lie down, if there is time
  - Making no attempt to restrain the person's movements or to put anything in his or her mouth
  - Moving away any object the person might hit, to protect the person from injuring him- or herself
- Maintain an airway by:
  - Loosening clothing, particularly around the neck

- Turning the person's head or body to one side so that saliva or vomitus drains out
- Opening an airway, if necessary, by lifting the person's shoulders and allowing the head to tilt back

If you find a person who is having a seizure:

- Do not leave the person.
- Do not move the person.
- Do not put anything in the person's mouth.
- Maintain an airway.
- Ring or call for assistance.
- Protect the person from self-inflicted injury.
- Watch the person carefully.
- Apply standard precautions when caring for a patient with seizure activity. There is a high probability of contact with blood, body fluids, secretions, and excretions during the care of this patient.

Nursing Assistant Care after the Seizure

When the seizure stops, tell the patient where she is and what happened. Assist her to bed. The patient will be very tired. Allow her to sleep. She may be confused and require periodic reorientation. Leave the patient in a position of comfort and safety with the call signal and needed personal items within reach. Other care includes:

- Providing incontinent care, if necessary
- Checking the vital signs as instructed; you may take vital signs frequently until the patient is stable
- Monitoring the patient closely for return of seizure activity
- Assisting the nurse to administer oxygen or suctioning, if needed

Report to the nurse:

- Any change in the patient before the seizure, such as an aura, confusion, or change in behavior
- A description of the way the seizure looked, including the body parts involved
- Loss of bowel or bladder control, eyes rolling upward, rapid blinking, biting tongue
- The time the seizure started and stopped, if known
- Condition of the patient after the seizure
- Vital signs

HUNTINGTON'S DISEASE (HD)

Huntington's disease (HD) is also called *Huntington's chorea.* This is a hereditary disease for which a genetic test is available. The test shows if individuals with a family history of the disorder have the gene. If the gene is present, development of the disease is inevitable. The disease is progressive and there is no cure. Disability and death occur within 15 to 20 years.

Signs and Symptoms

Clinical signs of HD usually begin when individuals are in their 40s or 50s, but in some individuals, symptoms may begin in childhood or young adulthood. Abnormal movements, called *chorea,* are the primary sign of Huntington's disease. The person appears anxious or restless, and seems to move frequently. The patient may try to disguise the activity with voluntary movements. As the disease progresses, rapid, jerking choreiform movements develop, involving the entire body. If the patient is ambulatory, he or she is at very high risk of falls. The person eventually loses voluntary control of all movement, as well as bowel and bladder control. The involuntary movement worsens if the person feels stressed or tries to control the choreiform motions.

Nursing Assistant Care

There is no known treatment or cure for HD. Aspiration, pneumonia, urinary tract infection and pressure ulcers often develop as the person deteriorates. The patient's response to pain and heat and cold sensitivity may be delayed. The nursing assistant monitors for sensation abnormalities and checks food and bath water temperature carefully. Goals of nursing care include:

- maintaining a consistent routine; avoiding changes as much as possible.
- keeping the patient as independent as possible for as long as possible.
- maintaining the person's current abilities.
- preventing weight loss and providing sufficient fluids.
- promoting safe swallowing, preventing choking.
- preventing falls and other injuries.
- maintaining the patient's ability to communicate.

Nursing assistant care also involves:
- supervising ambulation for safety.
- ambulating with a gait belt, if ordered.
- providing a recliner so the person can be out of bed.
- providing a seat belt when in the chair, if ordered.
- padding the siderails to prevent injury when in bed.
- giving the person as much control over daily routines as possible.

- treating the patient with dignity and respect.
- monitoring smoking behavior carefully.
- informing the nurse if you find smoking materials in a HD patient's room.
- avoiding insensitive remarks. Despite cognitive changes, the patients usually know what is going on around them.
- providing sufficient food and fluids. The movements will cause the patient to burn more calories and require more liquids.
- keeping mealtime as stress free as possible.
- allowing enough time for the patient to eat. You may have to reheat the food.
- assisting with feeding slowly, if necessary, while monitoring for choking and aspiration.

Persons with HD develop mental declines, which worsen over time. The person may be nervous, suspicious of others, and irritable. Mood swings and depression may occur. As the condition progresses, the individual develops dementia. He or she becomes totally dependent on others. Protecting the patient from falls and injuries is a high priority.

POST-POLIO SYNDROME

Post polio syndrome (PPS) is a neurologic condition marked by increased weakness and abnormal muscle fatigue in persons who had polio many years earlier. Estimates are that 30% to 70% of all polio survivors will develop this condition.

Nursing Assistant Care

- Provide reassurance and emotional support.

- Use nursing comfort measures, such as positioning and a backrub, to relieve pain.
- Inform the nurse of the patient's complaints of pain.
- Reduce strain and adjust activities to conserve energy.
- Provide a heat treatment to relieve pain, if ordered.
- Position comfortably in bed.
- Position to support weakened areas and deformities.
- Observe the patient's sleep at night and manage problems as they arise.
- Report your observations to the nurse.
- Encourage the patient to rest and nap periodically throughout the day.
- Help the patient pace activities and use measures to conserve energy.
- Position the patient as upright as possible during meals, and for 30 to 60 minutes after.
- Monitor the patient while eating and teach him or her to avoid talking while eating.
- Encourage her to alternate food and fluid and to avoid swallowing when the head is tipped back.
- Assist with oral care after meals to remove retained food particles.
- Monitor for dizziness when the patient stands up.
- If the patient complains of cold, provide socks or extra blankets.
- Caution the patient to call for help before getting out of the tub.

AMYOTROPHIC LATERAL SCLEROSIS

Amyotrophic lateral sclerosis (ALS) is a progressive neuromuscular disease that causes muscle weakness and paralysis. It affects the motor nerves that control voluntary movement. The cause is unknown. It is a progressive condition that is almost always fatal. In the United States, ALS is also called Lou Gehrig's disease.

Signs and Symptoms

Common signs and symptoms of ALS are:

- Stumbling, tripping, and falling
- Loss of strength and muscle control in hands, arms, and legs
- Difficulty speaking
- Difficulty swallowing
- Drooling
- Progressively more difficult breathing
- Muscle cramping, shaking, and twitching, progressing to spasticity
- Muscle weakness and atrophy
- Abnormal reflexes

ALS is not a painful disease, but the effects of ALS often cause pain. These are:

- Muscle cramps
- Contractures
- Constipation
- Burning eyes
- Swelling feet
- Muscle aches
- Pressure ulcers

ALS does not affect the entire body. The patient's mental acuity is intact. Depression is common. The heart is not affected, and bowel and bladder control and sexual function are not affected. The eyes are the last muscles affected and sometimes are not affected.

Nursing Assistant Care

Most patients with ALS are cared for at home, with brief hospitalizations to manage complications. Because of this, ALS is a family disease. Patients are taught to manage their own illness. Allow the patient to be in control of daily routines, and respect his or her intelligence. Adaptive equipment is used to maintain independence for as long as possible. Follow the patient's care plan for mobility. If the patient does not get out of bed, reposition and turn him or her at least every 2 hours, or more often.

Nursing care is designed to prevent complications of immobility. Care of the patient is largely determined by the progression of the patient's disease. Follow the care plan and nurse's instructions. Care of the typical ALS patient involves:

- Attention to positioning; an upright position (such as high Fowler's) may be ordered to ease respirations.
- Checking the skin carefully for signs of breakdown, and providing aggressive, preventive skin care.
- Following the care plan to manage the effects of spasticity, pain, and other potential complications, such as contractures.
- Range-of-motion and light exercise to prevent deformities and maintain strength of muscles that are not yet affected.
- Assisting the patient to use the incentive spirometer.
- Having the patient rest before meals to conserve muscle strength and reduce the risk of choking.
- Providing small, frequent feedings.
- Taking swallowing precautions when feeding the patient.
- Not washing solid foods down with liquids.
- Checking the mouth after meals to make sure there are no food particles that can cause choking later.
- Providing mouth care promptly after each meal.
- Scheduling rest and activities to preserve the patient's strength and energy.
- Using good infection control measures, hand washing, and standard precautions to reduce the risk of infection.

SPINAL CORD INJURIES

Injuries to the spinal cord result in loss of function and sensation below the level of the injury. Patients with such injuries are particularly prone to contractures and pressure ulcers. Special terms have been given to conditions resulting from such injury. These are listed in Table 13-1.

Signs and Symptoms

Signs and symptoms of paralysis vary with the level of the injury. The patient will be paralyzed below the level of injury to the spinal cord.

Responsibilities of the Nursing Assistant

Spinal cord injury patients need long-term nursing care, which includes:

- Listening. Many persons with spinal cord injury are taught to give directions to caregivers.
- A consistently calm and patient approach.
- Acceptance of the patient's expressions of anger, fear, and depression, as well as clumsy attempts at self-care.
- Careful skin care, because:
  - Incontinence not only causes the patient embarrassment and discomfort but also makes the skin prone to breakdown.
  - The lack of nervous stimulation decreases circulation to the skin.
  - Pain and pressure cannot be felt.
- Attention to elimination needs.
- Contractures and deformities occur rapidly after paralysis occurs. When moving and positioning patients with paralysis, move the extremities

Table 13-1	TERMS USED FOR DESCRIBING PARALYSIS

Paralysis is a complete loss of strength in an affected extremity or muscle group. Although rare, it may affect a single muscle. It commonly affects one entire region of the body. A pattern of weakness is a clue to identifying the origin of the nerve damage that is causing the paralysis. Paralysis affects voluntary movement, strength, and sensation.

- *diplegia*—paralysis affecting the same region on both sides of the body (such as both arms)
- *flaccid paralysis*—complete loss of muscle tone and absence of tendon reflexes.
- *hemiplegia*—paralysis on one entire side of the body (such as the arm and leg)
- *monoplegia*—paralysis affecting one limb only
- *paraplegia*—paralysis of the trunk (usually below the waist) and both legs
- *quadriplegia*—paralysis of the trunk (usually below the neck), both arms, and both legs (also see tetraplegia, below)
- *spastic paralysis*—movement of the affected muscles is spastic and not under the patient's voluntary control. The patient is aware of the spasms, but cannot stop them. This activity is much more severe than a common muscle spasm. *Spasticity* is usually strong and violent movement of an extremity without warning. It may be intermittent, frequent, or continuous. Spasms may be slow or rapid. They are often quite painful. Patients with upper motor neuron injuries and some neurologic conditions such as MS, ALS, and post-polio syndrome are most likely to experience spasticity.
- *tetraplegia*—another term for *quadriplegia;* the use of this word is encouraged, instead of using quadriplegia. The U.S. is the only country in which the term *quadriplegia* has been used. Medical personnel in other countries have always used the term *tetraplegia* to describe this condition. In 1991, The American Spinal Cord Association requested that medical professionals change the terminology to correspond with the terminology used elsewhere in the world.

slowly and gently. Rapid, rough movements will cause spasticity. If a patient's extremities move into a position of flexion, position them in extension. If the extremities move into a position of extension, position them in flexion. Positioning devices and splints may be necessary to maintain position.

- Range-of-motion exercises will be needed for the rest of the patient's life.
- Proper attention and care to prevent:
  - Respiratory infections
  - Urinary tract infections
  - Pressure ulcers

Autonomic Dysreflexia

Autonomic dysreflexia is a potentially life-threatening complication of spinal cord injury. It usually occurs in patients with injuries above the midthoracic area and indicates uncontrolled sympathetic nervous system activity. Problems that seem minor can trigger this condition. As a rule, injuries that would normally cause pain below the level of spinal injury can set this life-threatening chain of events in motion. Overfull bladder is the most common cause. Other problems that may trigger a crisis are:

- Urinary retention
- Urinary infection

- Blocked catheter
- Overfilled urinary drainage bag
- Constipation or fecal impaction
- Hemorrhoids
- Infection or irritation in the abdomen, such as appendicitis or acute abdominal conditions
- Pressure ulcers
- Prolonged pressure by an object in the chair, shoe, sitting on wrinkled clothing, and so forth
- Minor injury, such as a cut, bruise, or abrasion
- Ingrown toenails
- Burns, including sunburn
- Pressure on skin from tight or constrictive clothing
- Menstrual cramps
- Labor and delivery
- Overstimulation during sexual activity
- Fractured bones

Signs and symptoms of autonomic dysreflexia are:
- Extremely high blood pressure over 200/100 mm Hg
- Severe headache
- Red, flushed face
- Red blotches on the skin above the level of spinal injury
- Sweating above the level of spinal injury
- Stuffy nose
- Nausea
- Bradycardia
- Goose bumps below the level of injury
- Cold, clammy skin below the level of injury

If you observe any of these signs and symptoms, notify the nurse immediately.

Treatment for this condition involves identifying the offending stimulus and removing it. If you believe something has triggered the condition, inform the nurse. Remove tight and constricting clothing and shoes. Check the catheter and drainage bag. Follow the nurse's instructions.

MENINGITIS

Meningitis is an inflammation of the meninges. It is usually caused by microorganisms.

Sometimes this condition is treated with antibiotics. If it is communicable, droplet precautions are used.

CATARACTS

Cataracts are the leading cause of vision loss in adults over the age of 55. As a result, cataract surgery is one of the most common surgeries in the United States today.

Treatment

The latest innovations in cataract surgery are comfortable and convenient for the patient. The surgery is performed either as an outpatient procedure or in a day surgery center. The patient is admitted to the center in the morning and remains for 1 or 2 hours after the surgery, or until vital signs are stable.

Nursing Assistant Care

Nursing care of the cataract patient includes:
- Routine postoperative care.
- Relief of pain. Discomfort is mild. If pain is worsening, the patient complains of sharp pain, or if vision decreases, promptly notify the nurse.
- Being sure that all needed items, such as signal cords, are within easy reach.
- Taking extra precautions if the patient is confused or restless.
- Checking vital signs until stable.
- After surgery, the patient may feel as if something (such as an eyelash)

is in the eye. The patient may complain of itching. Slight fluid discharge may be present, and the eye may be sensitive to light and touch. Instruct the patient not to rub or squeeze the eye.

- The patient may complain of blurred vision. This is normal due to the bright lights used in surgery and drops used to dilate the eyes. The problem should resolve on its own promptly.
- Assist the patient with initial ambulation, if needed. Many patients are able to walk without help immediately after surgery.

After the patient is stable, he or she is usually discharged home.

GLAUCOMA

Glaucoma is a condition in which the pressure is increased within the eye. As the problem progresses, the patient begins to experience vision loss. If not treated, the patient will lose his sight.

Care of the Patient with Glaucoma

Care of the patient with glaucoma includes:
- Monitoring accurate intake and output if the patient is on intravenous medication to reduce eye pressure
- Checking vital signs every 2 to 4 hours
- Reporting complaints of eye pain promptly to the nurse
- Arranging needed items so the patient can see them; avoid moving things unless the patient gives permission
- Avoiding strain and exertion that will increase intraocular pressure
- Keeping the patient from stooping or lifting

- Avoiding tight and constrictive clothing, which also increases pressure
- Keeping the patient safe, if vision is limited

RETINAL DEGENERATION

Breakdown of the retina, known as retinal degeneration or *macular degeneration,* occurs over a period of months or years. The incidence increases with age. Central vision is progressively lost as the macula (area of acute central vision) is damaged.

NURSING ASSISTANT CARE OF THE PATIENT WITH A VISION IMPAIRMENT

The degree of visual limitation must be considered when giving care. It is also important to consider the patient's attitude toward the limitations. Adjustment to blindness is both a physical and an emotional process.

Allow the blind or nearly blind person the opportunity to do as much as possible in personal care and other activities. Most blind people do well with minimal help and support once they are fully oriented to their surroundings.

ARTIFICIAL EYE

Situations such as severe injury to the eye or untreatable cancer may require the surgical removal of an eye. An eye prosthesis (artificial eye) is usually inserted after the surgery. The care plan should provide information if the patient has an artificial eye. Some patients remove the artificial eye at night. You may be responsible for removing the eye. If the eye is to remain out of the socket, store it in a marked cup in contact lens disinfectant solution. The socket is usually cleansed and irrigated when the eye is removed. Apply the principles of standard precautions when caring for the artificial eye and mucous membranes in the eye socket.

WARM AND COLD EYE COMPRESSES

Many elderly patients have dry, itchy eyes. This may be caused by allergies, irritants, squinting, rubbing, or blinking the eyes. The eyes may appear red, with swollen eyelids. If patients rub or scratch their eyes, they may become infected.

Observe the patient for:
• Drainage from eyes
• Redness of eyelid rims
• Scaly, flaky skin around the eyes
• Edema of the eyelids

Report your observations to the nurse. You may be instructed to apply warm or cool soaks to the eyelids. Apply the principles of standard precautions when performing this procedure. If an infection is suspected, use separate equipment for each eye. This will prevent the infection from spreading.

HEARING IMPAIRMENT

Some of your patients will be hard of hearing or completely deaf. A hearing aid will sometimes improve the patient's level of hearing and comprehension. Lip reading or sign language may be needed to communicate.

Caring for Hearing Aids

A hearing aid is a delicate and expensive prosthesis. It requires safe handling and regular care.

Guidelines for Caring for a Hearing Aid

• Store hearing aids at room temperature when not being worn.

Temperature extremes can damage hearing aids. They should not be worn for more than a few minutes in very cold weather.

• Keep hearing aids dry. If an aid is worn accidentally in the shower, ask the nurse how to dry it. Never try to dry the aid with a hair dryer.

• Store extra batteries in a cool, dry place. Remove batteries from the hearing aid at night or open the battery compartment. This allows any moisture to evaporate.

• Keep hearing aids safe. They break easily if dropped on a hard surface.

• Remove the hearing aid if hair spray is being used, as the spray may cause damage.

• When an electric razor is being used, shave the patient before inserting the hearing aid, to avoid the noise from the electric razor being uncomfortable and annoying. Likewise, do not use a hair dryer when the aid is in place. The noise also is very uncomfortable for the patient, and the heat may damage the unit.

• Turn the hearing aid off when not in use. Turn the aid off before removing it.

• Wipe in-the-ear aids daily with a dry tissue.

• Check regularly to make sure the opening of the aid or earmold is free of wax. In-the-ear types come with a cleaning tool. This should be used only by someone who has been instructed how to use it. Never use a toothpick, paper clip, or other sharp object to clean the hearing aid.

• Insert the hearing aid properly. Sometimes the shape of the ear changes with aging and the hearing aid may need to be refitted. If the patient complains of pain or the aid is difficult to insert, this may be the problem. Advise the nurse if this occurs.

- When communicating with the patient, follow the same guidelines that you use when communicating with a hearing-impaired patient.
- Check the bed linen carefully before placing it in the soiled linen hamper. A hearing aid is small, expensive, and easily lost. It will not survive a trip through the washer and dryer!

Guidelines for Troubleshooting Hearing Aids

If the aid is not producing sound, before inserting it in the patient's ear:

- Check to make sure the "+" (positive) side of the battery is next to the "+" inside the hearing aid battery case or compartment. Hold the hearing aid in the palm of your hand. Turn the volume up all the way. Cup the aid between your hands. You should hear a loud whistle. A weak or absent sound indicates the battery is low. Try a new battery—the old one may be dead. Before changing the battery, check the position of the old battery so you can put the new one in the same way. When inserting a new battery, place it in the unit gently. If you meet resistance, do not force it. Consult the nurse.

- Check the earmold to see if it is plugged with wax.
- Make sure the hearing aid is set on "M" (microphone), not "T" (telephone switch).
- If the hearing aid works intermittently or makes a scratchy sound, check for dirt under and around the battery. Also check the volume control and connections. If the hearing aid has a connecting wire, make sure it is plugged in tightly and is not cracked or bent.

If the hearing aid is making squealing sounds:

- If the hearing aid is in the patient's ear and makes a loud, whistling sound, check the position. The aid should be securely in the ear. Make sure that hair, ear wax, or clothing is not interfering with the position. Check the tubing for cracks. Whistling usually indicates an air leak.
- Determine if the earmold fits properly. It should be completely in the ear. If it does not fit well, report it to the nurse.
- Check the volume on the aid. If it is too high, turn it down until the squealing stops.
- Check the plastic tubing on a behind-the-ear aid. If it is cracked or split, it must be replaced.

DISORDERS OF THE GASTROINTESTINAL SYSTEM

The tubelike mucous membrane structure of the alimentary canal lends itself to the possibility of malignancies, ulcerations, obstructions, and herniations.

MALIGNANCY

Treatment

Malignancies of the gastrointestinal tract are usually treated surgically by removing the affected part. For example:
- Esophagectomy—removal of the esophagus
- Subtotal gastrectomy—removal of part of the stomach
- Colectomy (bowel resection)—removal of part of the colon (large intestine)
- Colostomy—creation of an artificial opening in the abdominal wall and bringing a section of the colon to it for the elimination of feces
- Ileostomy—creation of an artificial opening in the abdominal wall and bringing a section of the ileum through it for the elimination of waste

ULCERATIONS

An ulcer (sore or tissue breakdown) can occur anywhere along the digestive tract. Common places are the:
- Colon—ulcerative colitis. In colitis, malnutrition and dehydration are brought about by loss of fluids in frequent, watery, offensive-smelling stools with mucus and pus.
- Stomach—gastric ulcer.
- Duodenum—duodenal ulcer.

HERNIAS

A hernia results when a structure such as the intestine pushes through a weakened area in a normally restraining wall. The danger of such abnormal protrusions is that some of the protruding tissue can become trapped in the weakened area. Circulation then becomes limited so that the tissue is in danger of dying. This is called an incarcerated (strangulated) hernia.

Frequent sites of herniation are:
- Groin area (inguinal hernia)
- Near the umbilicus (umbilical hernia)
- Through a poorly healed incision (incisional hernia)
- Through the diaphragm (hiatal hernia)

Hernias are usually repaired surgically with a procedure called a herniorrhaphy.

GALLBLADDER CONDITIONS

Two common conditions affecting the gallbladder are:
- Cholecystitis—an inflammation of the gallbladder
- Cholelithiasis—the formation of stones in the gallbladder. The stones may obstruct the flow of bile (fluid that aids digestion), causing:
  - Indigestion
  - Pain

– Jaundice (yellow discoloration of the skin and whites of the eyes)

Treatment

Cholecystitis and cholelithiasis may be treated by:
- Low-fat diet.
- Surgery to remove the gallbladder and stones. This surgical procedure is called a cholecystectomy.
- Laser therapy to break up stones.

Drains are often placed in the operative areas. Large amounts of yellowish green drainage may be expected.

In addition to routine postoperative care:
- Position the patient in a semi-Fowler's position.
- Do not disturb drains.
- If you notice fresh blood on the dressing, increased jaundice, or dark urine, report it immediately to your team leader.

COMMON PROBLEMS RELATED TO THE LOWER BOWEL

The frequency of bowel elimination varies with the individual. Some people have more than one bowel movement a day, but others have one every 2 or 3 days.

As foods move through the gastrointestinal tract by peristalsis, gas is formed. When the gas is expelled from the body, it is called "passing flatus," or flatulence. If the gas is not passed, it accumulates in the intestine. The abdomen will enlarge and appear bloated. *This is called abdominal distention and is an important observation to report to the nurse. Abdominal distention may also be caused by constipation and urinary retention.*

Observations to Make When Assisting Patients with Bowel Elimination
- You must observe the amount/quantity, color, odor, character, and consistency of the patient's bowel movement before discarding it.
- Notify the nurse if it has an unusual color, odor, or amount, or if the stool contains blood, mucus, parasites, or food particles (except corn and raisins). If you think a stool is abnormal, save it for the nurse to examine.

CONSTIPATION AND FECAL IMPACTION

Report problems with constipation to the nurse. The patient is probably constipated if he or she has not had a bowel movement in more than 3 days, strains, or passes hard, marblelike stools. Fecal impaction (Figure 14-1) is the most serious form of constipation. It is caused by retention of stool in the rectum, where it becomes hard and dry. The patient may be unable to pass it. The dried waste irritates the bowel. Mucus dissolves the hard, outer part of the mass. The rectum becomes so full that the fluid escapes around the impaction and is eliminated from the rectum as diarrhea. The patient may complain of:
- Abdominal or rectal pain
- Nausea
- Loss of appetite
- Feeling the need to have a bowel movement but being unable to do so

Other signs and symptoms of impaction are:
- Passing excessive flatus
- Bloating and abdominal distention
- Frequent urination
- Inability to empty the bladder
- Leaking around the catheter

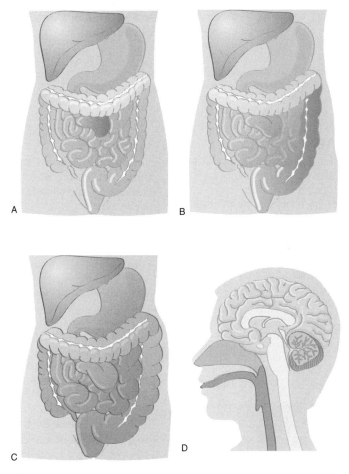

Figure 14-1 Progression of a fecal impaction, a life-threatening condition: (A) A fecal impaction blocks the rectum. The rectum and sigmoid colon become enlarged. (B) The colon continues to enlarge. (C) Fecal material gradually fills the colon. Digested and undigested food back up into the small intestines and stomach. The patient has signs and symptoms of acute illness, including lethargy, distention, constipation, and pain that is dull and cramping. (D) The entire system is full, and the patient vomits fecal material. The feces are commonly aspirated into the lungs.

- Mental confusion
- Fever
- Liquid stool or mucus seeping from the rectum

Fecal impaction is a very serious condition that is usually treated by manual removal of the mass by the nurse or advanced care provider.

Laxatives and enemas are also used to treat fecal impaction. The best thing to do is observe the patient's bowel elimination carefully and prevent fecal impaction from developing. Be conscientious in documenting patients' bowel activity and inform the nurse if a patient has not had a BM in 3 days or complains of discomfort.

DIARRHEA

Diarrhea occurs when peristalsis in the intestines is very rapid. The need to defecate is usually very urgent if the patient has diarrhea. Some patients may become incontinent because of the force with which the fecal material moves through the intestines. The patient may also complain of abdominal pain and cramping.

Undetected or untreated diarrhea can cause dehydration and other serious medical problems. Most health care facilities define diarrhea as having three or more loose stools within a specified period of time. One loose stool is not diarrhea. Remember to be objective in reporting your observations.

When reporting loose stools to the nurse, report the color, odor, consistency, character, amount, and frequency of stools. Also report any patient complaints of pain or other discomfort.

Role of the Nursing Assistant in Helping Patients with Bowel Elimination

Assisting with bowel elimination is a very important responsibility. Always apply the principles of standard precautions when assisting with elimination. Avoid contaminating environmental surfaces with your gloves. Wear a gown, eye protection, and face mask if splashing is likely.

Guidelines for Assisting Patients with Bowel Elimination

- Apply the principles of standard precautions when assisting with bowel elimination. Avoid environmental contamination with your gloves.
- Encourage patients to consume an adequate amount of fluid. Maintaining fluid intake is as important for bowel elimination as it is for urinary elimination.
- Encourage patients to eat a well-balanced diet.
- Allow adequate time for patients to eat meals.
- Encourage patients to chew food well. Cut it into small pieces if necessary. Report chewing problems to the nurse for further evaluation.
- If you observe a patient who has not eaten fiber foods, fruits, or vegetables, offer a substitute. The dietitian may visit the patient to discuss likes and dislikes and assure that he or she will eat the foods served.
- Encourage exercise and activity, as allowed and as tolerated.
- Assist patients with toileting at regular intervals and provide privacy.
- Position patients in a sitting position, if allowed, for bowel elimination.
- For privacy and warmth, use a bath blanket to cover patients using the bedpan or commode.
- Leave the call signal and toilet tissue within reach and respond to the call signal immediately.
- Allow adequate time for defecation.
- Provide perineal care as needed, or according to facility policy. Feces are very irritating to the skin, and prolonged contact promotes skin breakdown and infection.

- Assist patients with cleaning the anal area (this may be called the rectal area by some health care providers).
- Assist patients with hand washing and other personal hygiene after bowel elimination.
- Monitor bowel elimination and report irregularities.
- Record bowel movements on the flow sheet or other designated location. If a patient is independent with bowel elimination, ask if he or she has had a bowel movement each day.
- Report to the nurse: frequent stools, absence of stools, pain, cramping, excessive flatulence, abnormal color or consistency of stool, extremely small amounts of stool, hard, dry stool, or enlargement of the abdomen.
- Specific abnormalities in stools to report are presence of blood, pus, mucus, black or other unusual color, undigested food (except corn and raisins), or presence of parasites in the stool.

ENEMAS

A cleansing enema is the technique of introducing fluid into the rectum to remove feces and flatus (gas) from the colon and rectum.

The fluids often used for enemas are:

- Soap solution (SSE)
- Salt solution (saline)
- Tap water (TWE)
- Commercially prepared

General Considerations

Some general considerations to keep in mind are:

- If the patient is to get up following the enema and use the bathroom, make sure the bathroom is available

and not in use before giving the enema.

- When possible, the enema should be given before the patient's bath or before breakfast.
- Do not give an enema within an hour following a meal.
- Apply the principles of standard precautions. Avoid environmental contamination with your gloves.
- Administer an enema only upon the direction of a licensed nurse.
- Consult the care plan or the nurse for any special instructions and for the amount and type of solution to use.

Position

The best position for the patient to receive an enema is in the left Sims' position. Fluid flows into the bowel more easily when the patient is in this position. At times, the enema may have to be administered with the patient on the bedpan in the supine position. The supine position can be used if the patient is unable to hold the fluid or to assume Sims' position.

- The patient's knees are flexed and separated.
- An orthopedic (fracture) bedpan is more comfortable than a regular bedpan. It may have to be padded if the patient is very thin.

Giving an Enema with a Commercially Prepared Chemical Enema Solution

Commercially prepared enemas are convenient to administer and more comfortable for the patient. The enema may be either an oil-retention or a phosphosoda enema. The solution is already measured and ready to use.

- A small amount of fluid will remain in the container after administration.

• The solution in a commercially prepared enema draws fluid from the body to stimulate peristalsis.

• The oil-retention enema solution softens the feces, making them easier to expel.

• The amount of solution administered is about 4 ounces.

• The tip of the container is prelubricated.

• The enema solution is in an easy-to-handle plastic container.

• The solution is sometimes used at room temperature.

• You may be asked to warm the solution by placing the container in warm water before administration. Check with the nurse regarding your facility's policy.

Rectal Suppositories

Rectal suppositories are used to stimulate bowel evacuation or to administer medication. Medicinal suppositories must be inserted by the nurse. You may be asked to insert the type of suppository that softens the stool and promotes elimination. Check your facility policy to be sure this is a nursing assistant function. The suppository must be placed beyond the rectal sphincter (circular muscle that controls the anal opening) and against the bowel wall so it can melt and lubricate the rectum.

Rectal Tube and Flatus Bag

The rectal tube is used to reduce flatus (gas) in the bowel. Placing a rectal tube into the rectum provides a passageway for the gas to escape. Flatus distends the intestines, causing pain and stress on incisions.

You can assist the patient as follows:

• Encourage activity.

• Promote regularity.

• Accept the expulsion of gas as a natural body function. Do not contribute to the patient's embarrassment.

• Use flatus-reducing procedures when ordered.

• Insert a rectal tube with flatus bag if ordered. (Remember that your facility policies must state that nursing assistants can perform this procedure.)

The disposable tube is used once in a 24-hour period for no more than 20 minutes.

• Relief may occur as soon as the tube is inserted.

• Check the amount of abdominal distention (stretching).

• Question the patient about the amount of relief.

DISORDERS OF THE URINARY SYSTEM

Common conditions affecting the urinary system include inflammations caused by ascending or descending infections and obstructions to the normal flow of fluids through the tube structure.

CYSTITIS

Cystitis, or inflammation of the urinary bladder, occurs fairly frequently. It is particularly common in women because of the short length of the female urethra.

TREATMENT

Treatment is aimed at relieving the symptoms and eliminating the cause. Treatment includes:
- Bacteriostatic agents
- Increased fluid intake
- Antibiotics
- Monitor intake and output

NEPHRITIS

Nephritis means inflammation of the kidney.

TREATMENT

Treatment includes:
- Absolute bedrest
- Low-sodium diet
- Restricted food intake, at times
- Frequent checks on vital signs
- Accurate intake and output (I/O) measurement
- Steroid medication in some cases

RENAL CALCULI

Renal calculi are kidney stones. They can cause obstructions when they become lodged in the urinary passageways. There may be no sign of the development of renal calculi until an obstruction develops.

Treatment

The goal of treatment is to relieve the blockage and eliminate the stones.
- Encouraging fluids increases urine output. This helps to move the stones along the tract.
- All urine must be strained through gauze or filter paper, which is inspected for particles before it is discarded. Stones that are found can be analyzed. With information from the stones, the diet can sometimes be changed to make the formation of stones less likely.
- Monitor intake and output

NURSING ASSISTANT CARE OF THE PATIENT WITH A URINARY DISORDER

Be sure you understand the orders for each individual patient before you assist in nursing care. Orders regarding positioning, drainage, and activity for urological (urinary) patients vary.

Some important measures will apply to most urinary patients in your care:
- Accurately measure intake and output.

- Promptly report signs and symptoms of:
  - Bleeding
  - Chilling
  - Elevated temperature
  - Reduced output
  - Increased edema
  - Pain

- Properly care for urinary drainage.
- Know the proper steps to take for forcing fluids and for limiting fluids.
- When assisting with urination, collecting a urine sample, or recording intake and output, note and report the following:
  - Amount of urine
  - Color of urine
  - Odor of urine
  - Presence and type of sediment

URINE SPECIMENS

Routine Urine Specimen

Urinalysis is the most common laboratory test. The specimen is usually taken when the patient first voids (urinates) in the morning. Properties of fresh urine begin to change after 15 minutes. Therefore, it is important that you immediately take the sample to the laboratory or refrigerate it until delivery can be made.

Twenty-Four-Hour Specimen

If a 24-hour urine specimen is ordered, all urine excreted by the patient in a 24-hour period is collected and saved. Such a specimen requires that the patient start the 24-hour period with an empty bladder. For this reason, the first specimen is discarded.

- All urine is saved in a large, carefully labeled container that is supplied by the laboratory and may contain a preservative.

- The container is usually surrounded by ice. If the patient has an indwelling catheter, place the catheter drainage bag in a container surrounded by ice. Empty the bag into the container supplied by the laboratory.
- The patient is asked to void. This first urine is discarded so that the bladder is empty at the time the test begins.
- All other urine is saved, including that voided as the test time finishes.
- Toilet tissue should not be placed in the container.
- If you or the patient forgets to save a specimen during the test period, report it immediately to the nurse. The test must be discontinued and started again for another 24 hours.
- Remember to apply and remove disposable gloves each time you collect a specimen.

URINARY DRAINAGE

Many patients with urinary problems will be on urinary drainage.

- Urine is drained from the bladder through a tube called a catheter.

Sometimes the patient will complain of feeling the urge to urinate after the catheter is inserted. This is caused by the pressure of the balloon on the internal sphincter of the urethra. The pressure feels the same as the sensation of urine pressing on the sphincter.

If the patient with a catheter complains of feeling the urge to void, notify the nurse.

- A suprapubic catheter is inserted surgically through the abdominal wall directly into the bladder.
- A condom catheter is an external catheter used for males. It is applied over the penis and is attached to drainage tubing.

Nursing Assistant's Responsibilities

The nursing assistant has definite responsibilities when patients have urinary drainage:

- Apply the principles of standard precautions.
- Keep the urinary meatus clean.
- Wash the area around the meatus daily with a solution approved by your facility.
- Check regularly for signs of irritation or urinary discomfort and report them to the nurse.
- Secure the tubing so that there is no strain on the catheter or tubing. A catheter strap should be applied to the leg to secure the tubing.
- Maintain the drainage bag below the level of the bladder.
- When the patient is in bed, the closed drainage bag is attached to the frame of the bed, never the side rail.
- When the patient is in a chair or wheelchair, the closed drainage bag is attached to the frame of the chair.
- Many facilities use cloth catheter bags for visual privacy. The cloth bag is connected to the bed or chair frame, and the urinary drainage bag is placed in it.
- When the patient is ambulating, the tubing and drainage bag are carried below the level of the bladder.
- Secure the catheter with a strap or tape. When the catheter is secured to the leg, it is positioned on the top side. Avoid placing the catheter under the leg, which may pinch and obstruct the flow of urine. Know and follow your facility's policy.
- Attach the tubing to the bed with a rubber band and plastic clip.
- Use care when lifting, moving, and transferring patients with catheters to avoid accidentally dislodging the catheter by pulling on the tubing.

- Do not open the closed system.
- Make sure the tubing is not kinked or obstructed. Never attach it to the side rail.
- Ensure that the collection bag does not touch the floor.
- Measure the amount of drainage in the collection bag at the end of each shift, note the character of the urine, and report and record the information.
- In certain medical conditions, the physician will order an hourly output measurement. In this situation, a catheter drainage bag with a *urimeter* will be used. The urine drains into the small chamber. You will empty this chamber every hour, inform the nurse, and document the output measurement.
- Check the entire drainage setup each time care is given and at the beginning and end of your shift.
- Monitor the level of urine in the drainage bag. Most people excrete about 50 to 80 ml of urine each hour.
- If the level of urine in the bag does not change, if the catheter is leaking, if no urine is present in the bag, or if the urine has an abnormal color, odor, or appearance, inform the nurse.
- Notify the nurse if redness, irritation, drainage, crusting, or open areas are present at the catheter insertion site.
- Notify the nurse if the patient complains of pain, burning, or tenderness or has other signs or symptoms of urinary tract infection.
- When patients are ambulatory or using a geri-chair or wheelchair, you must be careful about the placement of the urinary drainage bag.
- Remember that the drainage bag must always be lower than the bladder so the urine cannot flow back into the bladder.

- The tubing must be secured to the patient's leg when the patient ambulates.
- When the patient is seated in a wheelchair, the tubing should run below and under the wheelchair so the drainage bag can be secured to the wheelchair back.
- The drainage bag or tubing must never touch the floor.
- At times it may be necessary to disconnect the catheter; follow your facility's policies for performing this procedure.
- In some facilities, a licensed nurse must give permission to disconnect a closed drainage system.

Infection Risk

The patient who has an indwelling catheter is at risk for infection. Infection can enter the drainage system at several sites:

- Urinary meatus, where the catheter is inserted
- Connection between the catheter and drainage tube
- Connection between the drainage bag and drainage tubing
- Opening used to empty the drainage bag

Disconnecting the Catheter

It is preferable to never disconnect the drainage setup, but at times it is necessary. If sterile caps and plugs are available, they should be used. If not, the disconnected ends must be protected with sterile gauze sponges.

External Drainage Systems (Male)

External urinary drainage systems are preferred for male patients who require long periods of urinary drainage. In external drainage, a catheter is not inserted in the urethra. Thus there is less danger of infection. Other complications, ranging from minor irritation to circulatory impairment can occur.

- The external catheter is applied over the penis. It is usually attached with an adhesive strip.
- *The strip should always be wrapped in a spiral. If it completely encircles the penis, severe injury can result.*
- Some external catheters have a self-adhesive film on the inside, making the adhesive strip on the outside unnecessary.
- About 1 inch of the catheter should extend beyond the tip of the penis and attach to the drainage tubing.
- Always apply the principles of standard precautions when caring for an external catheter.
- The condom is removed every 24 hours and the penis washed and dried.
- Inspect the condom catheter periodically to make sure it is not twisted or obstructed.

Leg Bag Drainage

Points to keep in mind when patients use a leg bag are:

- The leg bag is smaller than a regular drainage bag and must be emptied more often.
- The bag must be placed so there is a straight drop down from the catheter.
- Tension on the catheter tubing must be minimal.
- Take care to avoid introducing germs when connecting and disconnecting the closed drainage system.
- Avoid putting the patient to bed when wearing a leg bag.
- Disconnect the leg bag and connect the regular drainage bag when the patient is in bed.

DISORDERS OF THE REPRODUCTIVE SYSTEM

CHAPTER

16

PROSTATE CONDITIONS

Benign Prostatic Hypertrophy

- Prostate gland enlarges without tumor development
- Causes narrowing of the urethra, which passes through the center of the prostate gland
- Can produce sufficient enlargement to cause urinary retention
- Is noncancerous

Signs and symptoms of prostate conditions include difficulty in starting the stream of urine or in emptying the bladder completely.

Prostate Cancer

Prostate cancer is the second leading cause of cancer deaths in males. A blood test, the prostate-specific antigen (PSA), is used to screen for abnormalities.

Treatment

Various surgical approaches are used to remove all or part of the prostate gland (prostatectomy) to relieve urinary retention.

- Transurethral prostatectomy (TURP) —only enough of the gland is removed, working from inside the urethra, to permit urine to pass.
- Perineal prostatectomy—the entire gland is removed through surgical incisions in the perineum.
- Suprapubic prostatectomy—an incision is made just above the pubis and part of the gland is removed.

Male patients are likely to be disturbed by the necessity of having prostate surgery. Men often fear that they will not be able to have sexual intercourse after a prostatectomy. They feel that their manhood is threatened.

Urinary incontinence is also a common problem that is of great concern. In most cases, the rate of leakage decreases over time. Nevertheless, incontinence has a substantial impact on quality of life.

Nursing Assistant Care

The nursing assistant should:

- Wear personal protective equipment and apply the principles of standard precautions if contact with blood, body fluids, mucous membranes, or nonintact skin is likely.
- Make sure the tubes do not become twisted, stressed, or dislodged when positioning the patient.
- Carefully note the amount and color of drainage from all areas.
- Report at once any sudden increase in bright redness or the appearance of clots that seem to block the tube.
- Report to the nurse if dressings become wet with urinary drainage.
- Be patient and understanding of the patient's emotional stress.
- Refer questions about possible sexual limitation and urinary incontinence to the nurse so that the patient may be provided with accurate information and support.
- After prostate surgery, the patient may have a three-way catheter with a continuous irrigation.

- Inform the nurse if the bottle is low.
- Monitor the tubing for the presence of blood clots.
- Monitor the patient for signs of excess bleeding, cold clammy skin, pallor, restlessness, falling blood pressure, and rapid pulse. If such signs are noted, report them promptly.

CONDITIONS OF THE FEMALE REPRODUCTIVE ORGANS

Like the male organs, female reproductive organs are subject to disease processes, including tumors and infections.

Rectocele and Cystocele

Rectoceles and cystoceles are hernias. They usually occur at the same time.

- Rectoceles are a weakening of the wall between the vagina and the rectum. These hernias cause constipation and hemorrhoids (varicose veins of the rectum).
- Cystoceles are a weakening of the muscles between the bladder and the vagina. Cystoceles cause urinary incontinence.

Treatment and Nursing Assistant Care

A surgical procedure called colporrhaphy tightens the vaginal walls.

In addition to routine postsurgical care, you may assist in:

- Applying ice packs
- Giving sitz baths
- Giving vaginal douches (irrigations)
- Checking carefully for signs of excessive bleeding or foul discharge

Tumors of the Uterus and Ovaries

The most common indications of tumors of the uterus and ovaries are changes in the menstrual flow.

Treatment

Several types of procedures may be performed to treat tumors of the female reproductive tract, including chemotherapy, radiation, and surgery. Some surgical procedures are:

- Total hysterectomy—removal of the entire uterus, including the cervix.
- Oophorectomy—removal of an ovary. In younger women, at least a portion of the ovary is left to continue hormone production whenever possible.
- Salpingectomy—removal of a fallopian tube.
- Panhysterectomy—removal of the uterus and both ovaries and tubes. The surgical approach may be abdominal or vaginal. If a panhysterectomy is performed, the patient experiences surgically induced menopause. The more uncomfortable symptoms are sometimes relieved with hormone supplements.

Postoperative Care

In addition to usual postoperative care, the care following a hysterectomy will include:

- Caring for catheter drainage
- Possibly caring for a nasogastric tube, which may be in place to relieve abdominal distention and nausea
- Giving special attention to maintaining good circulation, because slowing of the blood supply to the pelvis may result in clot formation
- Introducing fluids and foods gradually after the initial nausea subsides
- Carefully observing the patient for low back pain
- Monitoring urine output and bleeding
- Checking both the abdominal incisional area and the vagina for presence and type of discharge
- Providing emotional support

TUMORS OF THE BREAST

Treatment

Mastectomy means removal of the breast. All or part of the breast tissue may be removed in a mastectomy.

- A simple mastectomy involves the breast tissue only.
- A radical mastectomy includes the breast tissue, underlying muscles, and the glands in the axillary area. This procedure is not performed as often as it was previously.
- A lumpectomy removes the abnormal tissue and only a small amount of the breast tissue.

Any form of mastectomy requires a great deal of psychological adjustment for the patient, who may have fear of disfigurement or fear of the loss of femininity.

Nursing Assistant Care

In addition to routine postoperative care, you will:

- Wear personal protective equipment and apply the principles of standard precautions if contact with blood, body fluids, mucous membranes, or nonintact skin is likely.
- Avoid taking the blood pressure on the side of the surgery.
- Monitor a blood transfusion as you would an intravenous infusion.
- Check pressure dressings frequently for signs of excess bleeding.
- Check the bed linen, because blood may drain to the back of the dressing.
- Report immediately numbness or swelling of the arm on the operative side.
- Be ready to offer support; walking may be difficult for the patient, who may feel unbalanced.

- Offer your fullest emotional support.
- Assist the patient in rehabilitative exercises.
- Refer questions about disfigurement and loss of femininity to the nurse.

SEXUALLY TRANSMITTED DISEASES (STD)

Sexually transmitted diseases (STDs) affect both men and women. Although most STDs can be treated and cured, patients do not develop immunity to repeated infections. It is possible to transmit the organisms causing STDs from:

- Mucous membrane to mucous membrane, such as from genitals to mouth or genitals
- Mucous membrane to skin, such as genitals to hands
- Skin to mucous membrane, such as hands to genitals

Using standard precautions correctly will protect the nursing assistant from contracting these diseases when caring for patients.

HUMAN IMMUNODEFICIENCY VIRUS (HIV) DISEASE

HIV disease is a viral disease. It is transmitted primarily through direct contact with the bodily secretions of an infected person. Therefore, it can be transmitted through direct sexual contact.

HIV disease destroys the immune system. There is no cure for this condition, although drugs can slow the damage to the body. If the disease progresses, the immune system is severely weakened. This stage of HIV disease is called acquired immune deficiency syndrome (AIDS).

CHAPTER

COMMUNICATION

17

As a nursing assistant you will need to receive and send information about your:

- Observations and care of patients
- Interactions with patients and visitors
- Patients' feelings

When communicating:

- Use a normal tone.
- Speak slowly.
- Use simple words.
- Look directly at the listener even if someone is interpreting.
- Try to obtain feedback from the patient to determine the level of understanding.

VERBAL COMMUNICATION

Choose words carefully so that your message is clear. Tone of voice, choice of words, and hand movements give clues to the real meaning of the message. Listen carefully to the message and watch the sender's facial expressions.

COMMUNICATING WITH PATIENTS

Message Interpretation

Always keep in mind how patients will interpret your message. We tend to think that the words we use are

Message Interpretation	
Your message is:	
Words	7%
Tone of voice	38%
+ Body language	55%
Total Communication =	100%

Figure 17-1 Your tone of voice and body language affect your message more than the words you use.

the most important part of the message, and this is not true. The nonverbal signals you send have a powerful effect on how others interpret the message (Figure 17-1). Keep this in mind when speaking with coworkers, patients, and visitors, and monitor your body language, tone of voice, and facial expressions.

COMMUNICATING WITH PATIENTS OF A DIFFERENT CULTURE

The patients you care for may come from many different cultures or have different ethnic backgrounds. Thus they may have unfamiliar customs, languages, and traditions. If you are assigned to someone from a different ethnic background, you should be given specific communication guidelines.

MEETING BASIC HUMAN NEEDS

DEALING WITH THE FEARFUL PATIENT

The experienced nursing assistant does not take remarks personally. The assistant realizes that the patient's complaints or refusal to cooperate may be a way of saying, "I need to be reassured and protected."

Give the patient an opportunity to talk. Listen carefully to everything that is said. You may be able to convince the fearful patient to assume some personal care whenever possible. If help in feeding, shaving, elimination, or other such personal matters is

needed, act in a very gentle, efficient manner and ensure the patient's privacy at all times.

To handle these situations successfully, the nursing assistant must:
- Recognize that this patient is a person with individual likes and dislikes.
- Give the quality of care that takes into account these likes and dislikes.
- Help the patient find ways to fill in time while in hospital. Boredom alone can lead to irritability.

Figure 18-1 shows the range of human needs. Needs on the lower

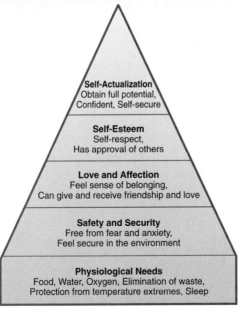

Figure 18-1 Maslow's hierarchy. The lower level needs must be satisfied before higher level needs become important.

level must be satisfied before the person can move to the satisfaction of the next level of needs.

Many personal problems affect the second level of the Maslow hierarchy. If a patient is anxious about a problem, such as how to pay the bills that accumulate while he or she is hospitalized, the anxiety over the unmet need may affect the patient's overall well-being. Some problems can seem so overwhelming that the patient appears distracted or consumed by them 24 hours a day. If a patient appears to be anxious about problems on the Maslow triangle, inform the nurse. Be a good listener. Allow the patient to talk about the problem, if desired, and provide emotional support.

GENERAL COMFORT MEASURES

ORAL HYGIENE

Oral hygiene is the care of the mouth and teeth. Patients requiring more frequent oral hygiene include those who are:

- Unconscious
- Vomiting
- Experiencing a high temperature
- Receiving certain medications
- Dehydrated
- Breathing through the mouth
- Receiving oxygen
- Receiving tube feedings
- Dying

BACKRUBS

When properly given, backrubs can be:

- Stimulating to the patient's circulation
- A major aid in preventing skin breakdown (pressure ulcers)
- Soothing
- Refreshing

Keep your nails trimmed to prevent injuring the patient. The backrub provides a good opportunity to observe the condition of the patient's skin. Report all observations to the nurse. Look for:

- Reddened areas that do not blanch (whiten) when pressed
- Raw areas of skin
- Condition of skin over bony prominences

Unless contraindicated, the backrub is given:

- Routinely as part of the bed bath or partial bath
- Following the use of the bedpan
- When changing the position of the helpless patient
- At bedtime
- When it could be comforting to the patient

Long, smooth strokes are relaxing. Short, circular strokes tend to be more stimulating. Avoid massaging red areas and over bony prominences. The backrub is given with warmed lotion.

COMFORT DEVICES

Footboard or Footrest

- Used to keep the feet at right angles to the legs (natural standing position).
- A footboard is always padded. It is used to prevent foot drop.
- If a footboard is not available, a pillow folded lengthwise may be placed against the foot of the bed to serve the same purpose.
- Special tennis shoes or soft boots may also be used to prevent foot drop in at-risk, bedfast patients.

Trochanter Roll

- The trochanter roll is used to prevent external rotation of the hips.

- Trochanter rolls should be used routinely for bedfast patients to prevent deformities.
- Unless a specific medical condition, such as hip fracture, is present, no special order is necessary. The roll can be made as follows:
  1. Fold a bath blanket lengthwise in thirds.
  2. Position patient in center of folded bath blanket. Blanket should extend from midthigh to above the waist.
  3. Roll each side of the blanket under and toward the patient until the blanket roll is firmly against the patient. Then tuck the roll inward toward the bed and patient to maintain the patient's position.

Pillows

Pillows are used to relieve pressure in such a way that spaces are left to relieve pressure in specific areas. This technique, called bridging, elevates an area of the body off the surface of the bed. It is useful for patients with healing pressure ulcers. Bridging is commonly used for the sacrum, hips, heels, and ankles. No special equipment is necessary. Facilities may use a combination of pillows, foam props, and bath blankets to support an area.

POSITIONING

COMPLICATIONS OF INCORRECT POSITIONING

The two most common complications are pressure ulcers and contractures. Pressure ulcers (bedsores) result when unrelieved pressure on a bony prominence interferes with blood flow to the area.

Contractures:

- Occur when a joint is allowed to remain in the same position for too long. The muscles stiffen and shorten (atrophy), making the joint incapable of full movement.
- Can begin to develop within as few as 4 days of immobility and inactivity. After approximately 15 days, the patient loses the ability to move the joint freely.
- Interfere with the patient's ability to move, complicate the provision of nursing care, and make treating pressure ulcers difficult.
- Cause bony prominences to suffer reduced blood flow. Some studies have shown a relationship between the presence of contractures and the development of pressure ulcers.

- Make movement and activity painful and difficult. Voluntary movement of the contracted joint becomes impossible as the contracture worsens.
- Can be prevented, and many can be reversed, with proper care.

Supportive Devices

Supportive devices are used to maintain proper body alignment and position in the bed or in a chair. They include:

- Pillows and/or folded sheets, bath blankets, or mattress pads to support the trunk and extremities.
- Splints and other specially designed orthotic devices (orthoses). Orthoses restore or improve function and prevent deformity.
- Special boots or shoes that are worn in bed to keep the feet in alignment.
- Bed cradles, which prevent pressure on the feet from the bed covers.
- Footboards to maintain foot alignment.

Contractures can be avoided by doing passive range-of-motion exercises consistently.

PATIENT POSITIONS

Figures 20-1 through 20-7 illustrate common positions.

Supine Position

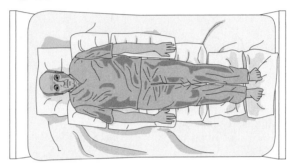

Figure 20-1   Supine position.

Semisupine Position

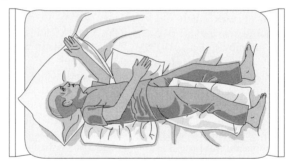

Figure 20-2   Semisupine position.

Prone Position

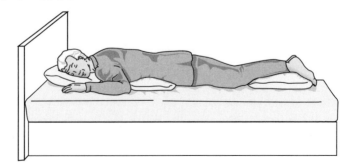

Figure 20-3   Prone position.

Semiprone Position

The semiprone position relieves pressure on the hips. Breathing is easier in this position than in the full prone position.

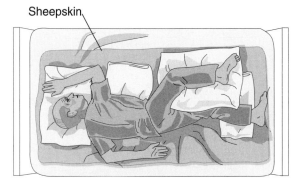

Figure 20-4   Semiprone position.

Right Lateral Position

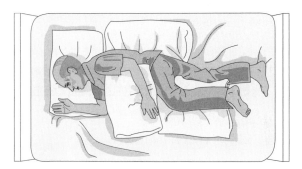

Figure 20-5   Right lateral position.

Sims' Position

This position is often used for rectal examinations, treatments, and enemas.

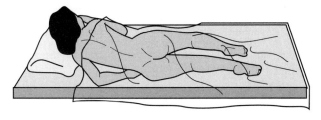

Figure 20-6   Sims' position.

Fowler's Position

This position is used for feeding patients in bed, for certain treatments and procedures, for the patient's comfort while visiting or watching television, and for those who are having trouble breathing.

The Fowler's position has a number of variations (Table 20-1). This is a common, comfortable position. Follow the care plan for the degree of head elevation and instructions for preventive skin care.

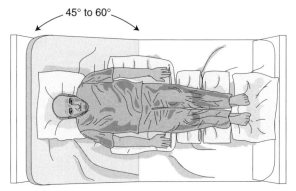

Figure 20-7   Fowler's position.

Table 20-1   FOWLER'S POSITION VARIATIONS

- *Low Fowler's position*—head of bed elevated 15° to 20° (degrees)
- *Semi-Fowler's position*—head of bed elevated 30° (degrees)
- *Fowler's position*—head of bed elevated 45° to 60° (degrees)
- *High Fowler's position*—head of bed elevated 90° (degrees)

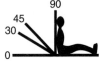

- *Orthopneic position*—head of bed elevated 90° (degrees) with the patient's shoulders back and chest fully expanded (Figure 20-8). The patient leans the upper body slightly forward and supports himself with the forearms. Used for patients with shortness of breath or difficulty breathing.

- *Tripod position*—similar to the orthopneic position. The head of the bed is elevated 90° (degrees) or as high as it will go. The patient can lift the arms and lean over a pillow or an overbed table (Figure 20-9), making it easier to expand the lungs fully. Used for patients with chronic lung disease, shortness of breath, or difficulty breathing.

Knee flexion may be used by elevating the lower end of the bed with the various Fowler's positions for patient comfort and to prevent sliding down in bed. Be aware that the Fowler's variations increase pressure on the coccyx, hips, and buttocks. Move the patient regularly and inspect the skin for redness or breakdown.

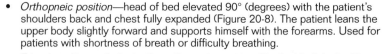

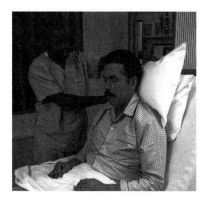

Figure 20-8   Orthopneic position.

Orthopneic Position

This variation of the high Fowler's position is used for patients who have difficulty breathing (Figure 20-8).

Sitting Position

Patients should be positioned in a comfortable, well-constructed chair so that the head and spine are erect. The back and buttocks should be up against the chair back. The feet should be flat on the floor. Refer to Chapter 8 for information on the 90-90-90 position.

REPOSITIONING

Changing a patient's position involves these steps:
1. Moving the patient into proper body alignment
2. Turning the patient onto the back, onto the abdomen, or to the side
3. Placing the patient's trunk and extremities in proper position and maintaining alignment with the use of supportive devices

Moving and Lifting Patients

• Always check the care plan or ask the nurse whether help is needed to lift or move a patient before proceeding with your assignment.
• Never be afraid to ask for help.

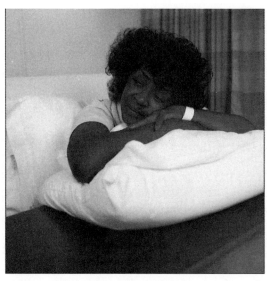

Figure 20-9   The tripod position enlarges the chest cavity, making breathing easier.

- By exercising caution, you are also preventing potentially serious injuries.
- Always check the care plan to see if there are special positioning instructions.
- A turning sheet or draw sheet (half sheet) may be placed under a heavy or helpless patient to make moving easier. The sheet must extend from above the shoulders to below the hips to be effective.
- Your back must last a lifetime. As a nursing assistant, many of the jobs you do increase your risk for back injury. If a mechanical device or other equipment such as a TLC pad (See Figure 28-1 of your book.) is available to use for lifting heavy items or moving patients, use it! Many new items have been developed in the last decade that make lifting and moving safer for both the nursing assistants and the patients. Spending a few minutes to retrieve the equipment is a worthwhile use of your time, and will help protect your back.

POSITIONING DEVICES

Several types of devices, often called splints, are used to maintain the position of an extremity. Their correct use prevents contracture formation.

Guidelines for the Use of Splints

- The splint must be applied correctly. Follow the manufacturer's directions.
- Follow the care plan for the patient's wearing schedule.
- Keep the extremity under the splint clean and dry.
- Keep the splint clean. If it becomes soiled, check with the nurse to see how it should be cleaned.
- Check the skin under the splint regularly for signs of redness, irritation, and skin breakdown.

PATIENT SAFETY

FALLS

Most incidents involving patients in any health care setting are falls.

Guidelines for Preventing Patient Falls

- Always leave the bed in its lowest horizontal position when you have finished giving care.
- Check to see whether the side rails are to be raised. Make sure they are attached securely.
- Check and adjust protruding objects such as bed wheels and gatch handles.
- Do not block or clutter open areas with supplies and equipment.
- Wipe up spills immediately.
- Encourage patients to use the rails along corridor walls when walking.
- Monitor patients for signs of weakness, fatigue, dizziness, and loss of balance.
- Monitor patients for safe practice if they independently:
  - Propel their wheelchairs
  - Transfer (get out of bed)
  - Ambulate (walk)
- Provide adequate lighting.
- Eliminate noise and other distractions that may increase confusion and create anxiety.
- Avoid leaving patients alone in the tub or shower unless you are given specific permission to do so.
- Check patients' clothing for fit and safety. Loose shoes and laces, long robes, and slacks increase the risk

of falling. Patients should wear footwear appropriate to the floor surface when walking and during transfers.

- Care for patients' physical needs promptly. Many incidents occur when patients attempt to get out of bed to go to the bathroom.
- Always use the correct techniques for transferring and walking patients.

USE OF PHYSICAL RESTRAINTS

Before the restraint is used, the staff must:

- Document all patient behavior that indicates a need for a restraint.
- Document all actions that were taken as alternatives to restraints.
- Consult with the patient and the family or legal guardian when alternatives are unsuccessful and obtain their approval and consent to apply a restraint.

Complications of Restraints

Complications of restraints are listed in Table 21-1.

RESTRAINT ASSESSMENT

- The care plan will provide information about the type of restraint to use, the time the restraint is to be applied, and other special information and instructions.

Table 21-1   COMPLICATIONS OF RESTRAINTS

POTENTIAL PHYSICAL PROBLEMS	POTENTIAL PSYCHOSOCIAL PROBLEMS
Decreased independence	Worsening of behavior problems
Pressure ulcers	Withdrawal, loss of social contact
Weakness	Depression
Decreased range of motion	Forgetfulness
Muscle wasting	Fear
Contractures (frozen, deformed joints)	Anger
Loss of ability to ambulate	Shame
Edema of ankles, lower legs, feet, fingers	Agitation
Decreased appetite, weight loss	Mental confusion
Dehydration	Combativeness
Acute mental confusion	Restlessness
Distended abdomen	Sense of abandonment
Urge to void frequently, dribbling	Frustration
Incontinence	Loss of self-esteem
Urinary tract infection	Screaming, yelling, calling out
Constipation	
Fecal impaction	
Lethargy	
Shortness of breath	
Pneumonia	
Bruising, redness, cuts, skin tears	
Falls	
Impaired circulation	
Blood clots	
Choking	
Death	

If restraints are indicated:
- The least restrictive restraint required to keep the patient safe should be selected.
- The restraint should be used as infrequently as possible.

Guidelines for the Use of Restraints

There are a few situations in which a patient may need a restraint, no matter how many alternatives are tried. When restraints are necessary, these guidelines must be followed:

1. A physician's order must be obtained by the nurse before restraints may be used. The order must indicate the type of restraint to use and the reason for its use. Try the least restrictive device first.

2. Use the right type and size of restraint. All restraints must be applied according to manufacturer's directions.

    Check the device before use— do not use if it is frayed, torn, has parts missing, or is soiled.

Restraints are put on over clothing, never next to bare skin. When applying a restraint to a female patient, make sure the breasts are not under the strap to the restraint.

3. Even if the patient does not seem to understand, always explain what you are doing. After application, check the fit of the device. You should be able to slip the width of three fingers between the restraint and the patient's body. The device should never restrict breathing.

4. The straps should be positioned so the patient is unable to reach them. The restraint straps should be smooth. Avoid twisting. Pad the restraint, if necessary to prevent irritation to the skin.

5. Tie restraint straps with slip knots for quick release in an emergency.

6. The patient should always have access to the signal light. Check every 15 minutes for the patient's comfort and safety. Make changes as needed.

7. When the patient is restrained in a wheelchair, the brakes should be locked when the chair is parked. The large part of the small front wheels of the chair should face forward. This changes the center of gravity of the chair and makes the chair more stable, preventing tipping.

8. Release the restraint at least every 2 hours for at least 10 minutes to:
   – Check for irritation or poor circulation
   – Change the patient's position
   – Exercise—ambulate the patient or do range-of-motion exercises
   – Take the patient to the bathroom
   – Change incontinent patients and cleanse their skin
   – Provide fluid or nourishment
   – Attend to any other needs
   Document each of these actions.

9. Maintain good body alignment whether the patient is in bed or a chair.

10. When restraints are used in bed:
    – There must be full side rails on the bed, in the up position.
    – The patient should always be positioned in the middle of the mattress.
    – Always secure the restraint to the movable part of the bed frame.
    – Make sure the straps are not at an angle when extended over the edge of the mattress. If the straps are angled even slightly, they will loosen if the patient moves up or down in bed.
    – Never tie the straps to the frame where the patient can reach and untie them. Fasten the straps in a slipknot to the inner springs, at least four inches in from the edge of the frame.

11. Do not use restraints in moving vehicles or on toilets unless you are sure the device is intended for that use by the manufacturer.

12. Gaps between the mattress and bed frame or rails can be caused by movement or compression of the mattress due to patient weight, movement, or bed position. If you observe a gap that is wide enough to entrap a patient's head or body part, inform the nurse promptly. Danger zones for patient entrapment are shown in Figures 21-1A and 21-1B. If potential entrapment is a problem, the bed can be modified with an

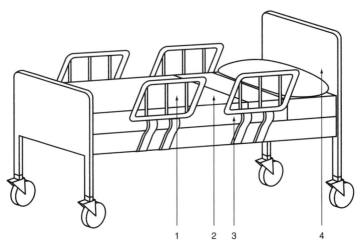

Figure 21-1A Entrapment between the mattress and side rails may occur: (1) through the bars of an individual side rail; (2) through the space between split side rails; (3) between the side rail and mattress; or (4) between the headboard or footboard, side rail, and mattress. (Courtesy of U.S. Food & Drug Administration.)

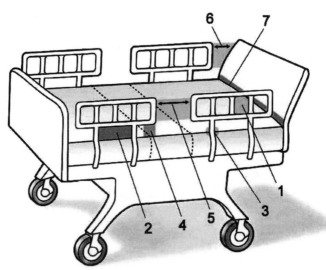

Figure 21-1B Zone 1: within the rail; Zone 2: between the top of the compressed mattress and the bottom of the rail, between the rail supports; Zone 3: between the rail and the mattress; Zone 4: between the top of the compressed mattress and the bottom of the rail, at the end of the rail; Zone 5: between the split bed rails; Zone 6: between the end of the rail and the side edge of the head or foot board; Zone 7: between the head or foot board and the mattress end. (Courtesy of U.S. Food & Drug Administration.)

adaptive device or another bed can be used or the mattress modified to prevent injury.

Other observations that will help eliminate the need for restraints are:

- Does the patient see and hear well? Does the patient normally wear glasses? Is he or she wearing them now? Are they clean? Does the hearing aid work? Are the patient's ears plugged with wax? Sometimes behavior problems, balance problems, and other safety problems are caused because the patient is out of touch with the environment. Applying these simple corrective devices may eliminate the need for a restraint.
- Is the patient able to make her needs known? Sometimes unsafe behavior is caused by an unmet need. Discovering this need and meeting it may help you avoid using a restraint.
- Does noise or confusion in the environment cause the patient to become agitated? Noise can be caused by other patients or staff, the public address system, radios, or television. Eliminating the noise may stop the behavior.

- Does the behavior occur during a certain time of day, during a certain activity, or when a specific person is providing care?
- Does the patient seem uncomfortable? Physical pain, hunger, thirst, or the need to use the bathroom can cause unsafe behavior.
- Does the patient seem lonely or isolated? Bored? Boredom, loneliness, or looking for a misplaced item can cause unsafe behavior.
- Does the patient try to get out of bed or a chair without help? Is the patient steady on his or her feet? Does he or she normally use a cane or walker? Is he or she using it now? Is the call signal available, and does the patient know how to use it? Would the patient benefit from use of an alarm that sounds when he or she stands up? Would use of an alarm remind the patient to sit down, alert the staff, and eliminate the need for a restraint?

If you make an observation of a condition that causes confusion or agitation, or discover an approach that is effective in eliminating or reducing the need for restraints, inform the nurse.

REST AND SLEEP

SLEEP

Signs and symptoms of inadequate sleep are:
- Slow mental and physical responses
- Decreased attention span
- Forgetfulness, difficulty remembering things
- Reduced reasoning and judgment
- Puffy, red, swollen eyes
- Dark circles under eyes
- Disorientation
- Mood swings, moodiness
- Lethargy, sleepiness, fatigue
- Agitation, restlessness
- Clumsiness, incoordination
- Difficulty finding the right word(s) to say
- Slurred speech
- Hallucinations in severe sleep deprivation

Nursing Measures to Promote Rest and Sleep

Basic nursing measures may make the patient more comfortable and promote rest and sleep. These include:
- Tell patients what you are doing and how you will do it.
- Handle the patient gently during care. Avoid sudden, jerking movements when moving or positioning the patient.
- Use pillows to support the affected body part.
- Maintain a comfortable environmental temperature.

- Provide extra blankets or pillows as needed.
- Assist the patient to put on comfortable clothing for rest and sleep.
- Eliminate unpleasant odors.
- Assist the patient with toileting or with incontinence care.
- Avoid startling the patient.
- Eliminate or reduce noise.
- Work quietly in the hallways, handle equipment carefully, speak in a low voice with coworkers, and limit conversation.
- Organize care to allow the patient uninterrupted sleep or rest.
- Eliminate pain, such as offering a backrub or assisting the patient to assume a comfortable position.
- Report pain to a licensed nurse.
- If a patient is having pain, wait for at least 30 minutes after administration of pain medication before performing procedures.
- If a patient is anxious, listen to what he or she says; eliminate the cause of anxiety, if possible.
- Play soft music to distract the patient.
- Avoid physical activity or other activities that are upsetting to the patient before bedtime.
- Assist the patient to perform bedtime rituals, if any.
- Allow the patient to select his or her own bedtime.
- Provide a warm bath or shower, if preferred.

- Avoid serving beverages containing caffeine before bedtime.
- Provide a bedtime snack, if desired.
- Allow the patient to read, watch television, or listen to the radio, if desired.
- Read to the patient from a favorite book.
- Assist with relaxation exercises and activities, as ordered.
- If the patient receives a sleeping medication, make sure he or she is ready for sleep when the nurse administers the medication.
- Listen to the patient's concerns.
- Provide emotional support.
- Adjust lighting to a comfortable level for the patient; darken the room as much as possible for sleep.
- Keep bed linen clean and wrinkle free.
- Offer food or beverage.
- Meet the patient's physical needs.
- Close the door to the patient's room.

Sleep Needs

Table 22-1   SLEEP NEEDS ACROSS THE LIFE SPAN
Newborn infants sleep in 3- to 4-hour intervals for a total of 16 to 20 hours of sleep per day.
Infants require 12 to 16 hours of sleep per day.
Toddlers require 12 to 14 hours of sleep per day, usually broken down into 10 to 12 hours of sleep at night, with one or more daytime naps.
Preschool children require 10 to 12 hours of sleep per day.
Elementary school children require 10 to 12 hours of sleep per day.
Adolescents require 8 to 10 hours of sleep per day.
Young adults aged 18 to 40 require about 7 to 8 hours of sleep per day.
Middle-aged adults aged 40 to 65 require about 7 hours of sleep per day.
Elderly adults over age 65 require about 5 to 7 hours of sleep per day.

EMPHASIS ON NOISE CONTROL

Comfort, rest, and sleep are important for patient well-being. Excessive noise has been shown to delay healing, impair immune function, and increase heart rate and blood pressure. Patients may feel very stressed or anxious, and may not realize the noise is the cause of their distress. Patients who do not sleep well at night may be unhappy with care and be unable to stay awake during the day for meals and therapy. Some patients become confused and agitated when sleep deprived. Confused patients may begin wandering to escape the noise.

The Occupational Safety and Health Administration (OSHA) has established noise standards for employee safety. Under these standards, workers should not be exposed to 90 decibels of sound for more than eight hours. The Environmental Protection Agency (EPA) recommends that hospital noise levels should not exceed 45 decibels during the day. During one study, decibel levels as high as 113 were recorded at night. Noises that were tolerable during the day were more disruptive at night.

An uncomfortable noise level has been called an invasion of privacy by some patients. This is a concern, because the patient is powerless to control the noise that is disturbing him or her. Noise should never interfere with the patients' ability to hear, cause patients distress or anxiety, or make patients feel as if the noise is an invasion of their privacy.

In addition to adversely affecting patients, excess noise causes extra stress and fatigue for staff. Having to talk louder and having to be more attentive when listening to others is considered one of the leading causes of fatigue in hospital staff. Do all that you can to control sources of unnecessary or excessive noise. Follow your facility policies and do all you can to reduce noise when you are on duty.

PAIN

PAIN:

- Is never normal. It is always a warning that something is wrong.
- Interferes with the patient's optimal level of function and self-care.
- Causes patients to limit movement.
- When unrelieved, contributes to periods of immobility, increasing the risk of pneumonia, skin breakdown, and other problems.
- Decreases the quality of life and may cause anxiety, depression, and a feeling of helplessness.
- May cause acting out, crying, and other strange, belligerent, or combative behavior.

IDENTIFYING PATIENTS IN PAIN

- Many facilities now consider pain the "fifth vital sign." In these facilities, pain is regularly and frequently evaluated.
- Always report patient complaints of pain to the nurse, describing the pain in the patient's exact words.
- Be very factual in reporting observations of pain and behavior.
- Always report verbal complaints of pain. Never try to judge whether a patient really has pain or how severe it is.
- Never compare patients. One person may seem to be in more pain than another person with the same diagnosis. It is not appropriate to

think that they should both respond in the same way.
- Body language is often the first clue that a patient is having pain. This is particularly true with pediatric and cognitively impaired patients, those from other cultures, and patients who are comatose.
- Look for pain on movement, facial expressions, crying, moaning, rigid posture, and guarded positioning. The patient may withdraw when he or she is touched or repositioned. Watch for restlessness, irregular or erratic respirations, intermittent breath holding, dilated pupils, and sweating. The patient may favor one extremity. He or she may become irritable, fatigued, or withdrawn. The patient may refuse to eat, for no apparent reason.
- Always suspect pain if the patient's behavior changes.
- Although the patient may not display an outward appearance of pain, asking if he or she is having pain is the best way to find out.
- Regularly ask patients if they are in pain. Some will not volunteer this information if not asked directly.
- When asking patients about pain, make sure the patient can see and hear you. Allow enough time for the patient to process your questions and respond. Be patient. Use language that is appropriate for the patient's age and mental status.

- Whatever is painful for adults also will be painful for children, perhaps more so.
- Report your observations to the nurse compared with the normal behavior for the patient.
- If the behavior changes back to normal after the nurse administers an analgesic (pain) medication, this confirms that the change in body language or behavior was caused by pain.
- The patient's self-report is the most accurate and reliable indicator of pain and should be believed and respected.
- Avoid passing judgment on patients who take narcotic analgesic medications to control their pain. Many health care workers try to discourage patients from taking these drugs because of the potential for addiction. Studies have shown that very few patients with severe pain become addicted to the drugs.
- The nurse may use a pain scale to help assess and manage the patient's pain. Become familiar with the scales used at your facility.
- If a patient has been medicated for pain but continues to complain, report this information to the nurse. Do not assume the pain has been relieved after a medication has been given, even if the patient is laughing or talking. Ask the patient. If he or she admits to continued pain, the nurse must evaluate the patient further.

Other important information you may see, hear, and observe that should be reported to the nurse includes:
- Vital signs
- Skin color
- Location of pain (specific site of pain on the body)
- Radiation, if any (movement of pain to other areas)

- Time of onset (when the pain began)
- Duration (how long the pain lasts)
- Frequency (how often it occurs)
- Pain quality (nature and type of pain)
- Pain intensity (strength and description of pain, in the patient's own words)
- Aggravating and alleviating factors (things that improve or worsen the pain)
- Character (properties, features, characteristics)
- Variation or patterns of pain (changes in pain or cycles of pain)
- Pain management history, if any (things the patient tells you about past history of pain and things that make it better or worse)
- Present pain management regimen, if any, and its effectiveness (things the patient does to relieve pain, including response to comfort measures and medications)
- Effect of pain on activities of daily living, sleep, appetite, relationships, emotions, concentration, and so forth
- Direct observation of abnormalities at the site of the pain
- Other observations, such as facial expressions, body language, movements, nausea, or vomiting
- Side effects of analgesic (pain-relieving) medications, if applicable
- Response to pain medications and other forms of treatment, if applicable

USING A PAIN RATING SCALE

Using a pain rating scale helps nurses evaluate the patient, helps prevent subjective opinions, provides consistency, and gives the patient a means to describe the pain accurately (Figures 23-1A–G).

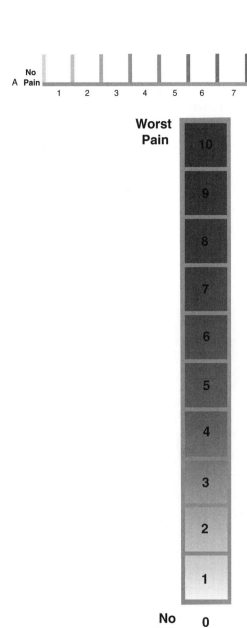

Figure 23-1A–B   (A) Horizontal numeric pain scale. (B) Vertical numeric pain scale.

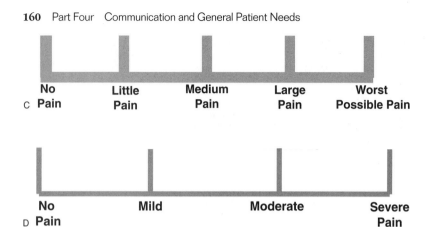

| No Pain | Little Pain | Medium Pain | Large Pain | Worst Possible Pain |

C

| No Pain | Mild | Moderate | Severe Pain |

D

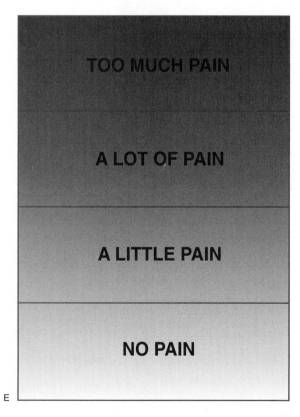

E

Figure 23-1C–E   (C) Verbal descriptor pain scale. (D) Verbal pain scale. (E) Verbal pain scale.

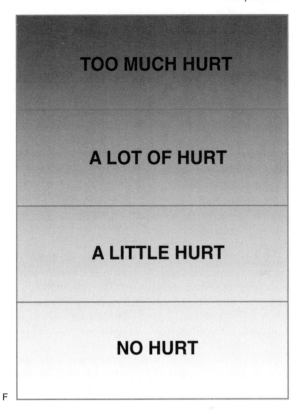

TOO MUCH HURT

A LOT OF HURT

A LITTLE HURT

NO HURT

F

G Alternate
   Coding

0	1	2	3	4	5
NO HURT	HURTS LITTLE BIT	HURTS LITTLE MORE	HURTS EVEN MORE	HURTS WHOLE LOT	HURTS WORST
0	2	4	6	8	10

Figure 23-1F–G (F) Verbal pain scale. (G) The FACES scale is excellent for children and adults, as well as patients who do not speak English. (FACES Pain Rating Scale from Hockenberry MJ, Wilson D, Winkelstein ML: *Wong's Essentials of Pediatric Nursing,* ed. 7, St. Louis, 2005, p. 1259. Used with permission. Copyright, Mosby.)

MANAGING PAIN

- Notify the nurse as soon as the patient complains.
- Report your observations objectively.
- Observe the patient carefully after medications have been given and report your observations to the nurse.

Nursing Comfort Measures

- Telling patients what you plan to do and how you will do it
- Providing privacy
- Assisting the patient to assume a comfortable position, repositioning the patient for comfort to relieve pain and muscle spasms, changing the angle of the bed to relieve tension on surgical sites or injured areas
- Avoiding sudden, jerking movements when repositioning the patient
- Performing passive range-of-motion exercises to reduce stiffness and maintain mobility

- Using pillows to support the affected body part(s)
- Providing extra pillows for comfort and support
- Straightening the bed and linen
- Giving a backrub
- Washing the patient's face and hands
- Providing a cool, damp washcloth on the patient's forehead
- Providing oral hygiene
- Providing fresh water, food, or beverages as permitted
- Playing soft music to distract the patient
- Listening to the patient's concerns
- Providing emotional support
- Maintaining a comfortable environmental temperature
- Providing a quiet, dark environment
- Eliminating sources of unpleasant sights, sounds, and odors from the environment
- Waiting at least 30 minutes after the nurse administers pain medication before moving the patient, performing procedures, or activities

LIFE SPAN DEVELOPMENT

NEONATE

- Has a large head that seems disproportionate the body.
- Has wrinkled, thin, red skin.
- Appears to have a protruding abdomen.
- Has dark blue eyes.
- Has uncoordinated movements.
- Does not have clear vision, but hearing and taste are developed.
- Has developed certain reflexes:
  - Moro reflex—a loud noise startles the infant, causing it to spread the arms, extend the legs, and thrust back the head.
  - Grasp reflex—touching the infant's palm causes the fingers to flex in a grasping motion.
  - Rooting reflex—stroking the cheek or side of the lips stimulates the infant to turn its head in the direction of the stroking.
- Diet is milk or milk substitute.
- Routine is largely sleeping, eating, and eliminating.
- Is completely dependent on the caregiver for all needs.
- Is unable to support her head, so must be handled carefully and be well supported when held.

THREE-MONTH-OLD INFANT

- Has gained enough muscular coordination to hold up his or her head and raise the shoulders.

- Has lost the Moro, rooting, and grasp reflexes.
- Produces real tears.
- Can follow objects with his eyes.
- Can smile and coo at the caregiver.

SIX-MONTH-OLD INFANT

- Has learned to roll over.
- Can sit for short periods of time.
- Holds things with both hands and then directs them toward his or her mouth.
- Responds with verbal sounds when a caregiver speaks.
- Is beginning to cut front teeth.
- Eats finger foods and strained fruits and vegetables.
- Recognizes family members.
- Develops fear of strangers.

NINE-MONTH-OLD INFANT

- Crawls and may begin to stand when supported.
- Has more teeth erupt.
- Can respond to his or her name.
- Says one- and two-syllable words such as "mama."
- Shows a preference for right or left hand control.
- Eats junior baby foods.

ONE-YEAR-OLD INFANT

- Understands simple commands such as "No."
- Begins to take steps—supported at first, then independently.
- Eats table foods and can hold a cup.

- Weighs three times what he or she weighed at birth.

TODDLER

(2 to 3 years)
- Learns to control elimination.
- Begins to become aware of right and wrong.
- May react with frustration to attempts at socialization and discipline with increased awareness of him- or herself as a separate person.
- Tolerates brief periods of separation from the mother, but the mother remains the source of security and comfort.
- May play in the company of other children but with no interaction. "No" and "mine" are a major part of their vocabularies.

At the end of this period, the toddler is able to:
- Walk and run.
- Display motor (manual) skills that include feeding self and riding toys.
- Put words together and speak more clearly. The average vocabulary is about 300 words.
- Play near others, but is not able to interact in play with children of the same age (peers).

PRESCHOOL CHILD

(3 to 5 years)
- Grows less reliant on the mother. Begins to recognize own position as a member of the family unit and own uniqueness from other family members.
- Develops rivalries with siblings and develops greater attachments to the father or alternate caregiver.
- Gradually increases cooperative play.
- Improves language skills and asks many questions.

- Develops a more active imagination.
- Becomes more sexually curious.

SCHOOL-AGE CHILD

(6 to 12 years)
- Is able to communicate.
- Has developed small (fine) motor skills. With these skills, the child is able to master tasks such as writing.
- Develops an increased sense of self.
- Establishes peer relationships.
- Reinforces proper social behavior through games, simple tasks, and play.
- Chooses sex-differentiated friends.
- Joins groups like Boy Scouts or Girl Scouts. This serves to further identify the individual as a person of a particular gender.
- Begins to show concern for other living things.

PREADOLESCENT

(12 to 14 years)
- Hormonal changes stimulate the secondary sex characteristics.
- The individual feels on the threshold of tremendous change, though not yet in a period of sexual functioning.
- Mood swings and feelings of insecurity are common.
- There is a growing awareness of and interest in the opposite sex.
- Arms and legs seem out of proportion to the rest of the body.

ADOLESCENT

(14 to 20 years)
- Gradual development of sexual maturity.
- A greater appreciation of the individual's own identity as a male or female person.

- Conflicting desires for the freedom of independence and the security of dependence. As a result, this is often a troublesome period.
- The establishment of personal coping systems and the ability to make independent judgments and decisions.
- Gradual success in mastering developmental tasks of the age. The adolescent is able to make comparisons between the values she has been taught and reality.

ADULTHOOD

(20 to 50 years)
- Independence and decision making.
- The choice of a mate.
- Establishment of a career and family life.
- Optimal health.
- The choice of friends to form a support group.

MIDDLE AGE

(50 to 65 years)
- Final career advancement, ending in retirement.
- Children who were reared during the period of adulthood leaving home to enter their own adult period.
- Health that is usually still at good levels, though some slowing may be seen.
- More time that can be spent on leisure activities.
- More time and money to pursue personal interests.

- Revitalizing one's relationship with a mate.
- Enjoying grandchildren.
- For some middle-aged persons, being a member of the "sandwich" generation—caring for both their own parents and their children or grandchildren.

LATER MATURITY

(65 to 75 years)
- A gradual loss of vitality and stamina.
- Physical changes that signal the aging process. For example, sight and hearing diminish.
- Chronic conditions that develop and persist.
- A period of gradual losses: loss of mate, friends, self-esteem, some independence.
- Examination of a lifetime.
- More time to pursue personal interests.
- Fewer responsibilities related to raising a family and holding a job.
- Increased wisdom.

OLD AGE

(75 years and beyond)
- Failing physical health and growing dependency.
- The need to deal with illness, loneliness, loss of friends and loved ones, and the realization of mortality. Success in this period depends on the mechanisms of coping developed in earlier years.

DEVELOPING CULTURAL SENSITIVITY

25

Consider the ways in which your patient's culture may influence the way you provide care:

- It may not be acceptable to discuss personal matters before developing rapport with the patient.
- Discussion of sexual matters with the opposite sex might be considered taboo.
- The patient may agree with what you say just to be polite, without really understanding the conversation. Ensure that he or she understands by asking questions.
- Any casual physical contact might be forbidden. Find out what sort of touch is appropriate.
- The patient may be extremely modest.
- Direct eye contact might be considered impolite.
- Gestures might have different and offensive meanings.

- The decision maker in the patient's culture may be someone other than the patient, such as a mother or husband.
- Some foods and beverages might be considered taboo.
- The patient might have different hygiene standards.
- The patient may find it difficult to accept instructions from a woman.
- The patient might have a different concept of time.
- The patient may believe illness is caused by something supernatural, such as black magic.
- The patient might respond to pain differently—with stoicism, or with a lot of noise.
- There might be a different attitude toward dying and death.
- Some days might be considered sacred, and the patient may refuse to accept care during prayer time.

PERSONAL SPACE

Table 25-1 CULTURAL INTERPRETATION OF NONVERBAL COMMUNICATION AND PERSONAL SPACE

CULTURE	NONVERBAL COMMUNICATION
American (U.S.)	Personal space of 18 to 36 inches. Eye contact is acceptable. Lack of eye contact may be interpreted as lack of self-esteem or not telling the truth.
African American	Eye contact is acceptable. Close personal space.
Arab American	Women usually avoid eye contact with men and others whom they do not know well. Close personal space.
Asian	Varies by country; most consider eye contact disrespectful. Close personal space, but avoid touching.

Table 25-1	CULTURAL INTERPRETATION OF NONVERBAL COMMUNICATION AND PERSONAL SPACE (CONTINUED)

CULTURE	NONVERBAL COMMUNICATION
Brazilian	Lack of eye contact is viewed by some as a sign of respect. Close personal space.
Cambodian	Eye contact is acceptable. Close personal space.
Chinese American	Avoid eye contact with authority figures as a sign of respect; will make eye contact with family and friends. Distant personal space.
Colombian	May avoid eye contact in presence of an authority figure. Close personal space.
Cuban	Eye contact expected during conversation. Close personal space with friends and family.
Ethiopian	Avoid eye contact with those perceived to be in authority. Close personal space with family and friends.
European	Eye contact acceptable. Distant personal space.
Filipino	May avoid eye contact with authority figures. Close personal space.
Gypsy	Facial expressions reflective of mood. Close personal space with family members. This group generally avoids contact with non-Gypsies. Also avoids surfaces considered unclean (areas that lower body has touched).
Haitian	Avoid eye contact with those perceived to be in authority.
Hmong	Avoid prolonged eye contact, which is considered rude.
Iranian	Make eye contact only with equals and close family and friends. Close personal space.
Japanese American	Little eye contact. Touching may be considered offensive.
Korean	Make little direct eye contact. Touching considered offensive. Although Koreans maintain close personal space with family, invading their personal space is a sign of disrespect.
Mexican American	Avoid eye contact with those perceived to be in authority. Some may believe touch by strangers is disrespectful or offensive.
Native American	Eye contact avoided as a sign of respect. Distant personal space is considered respectful.
Puerto Rican	Personal space varies with age-group; generally closer with younger women, more distant with older women.
Russian	Direct eye contact acceptable during conversation. Close personal space with family and friends.
South Asian	May consider direct eye contact with elderly individuals offensive or rude. Close personal space with family members.
Vietnamese	Avoid eye contact with those perceived to be in authority. Distant personal space.
West Indian	Eye contact is avoided. Distant personal space.

BELIEF SYSTEMS

Table 25-2 BELIEF SYSTEMS RELATED TO HEALTH/ILLNESS

CULTURE	RELATED CONCEPTS	HEALTH CARE PROVIDER	CAUSE OF ILLNESS	METHODS OF TREATMENT
European Americans	Illness can be influenced by poor health practices; disease is treatable and sometimes curable	Physician	• Punishment for sins • Self-abuse; outside forces such as germs	Diet, exercise, home remedies, medication, surgery, religious rituals, wearing amulets
Asian Americans	Body has two energy forces: *yang*, which is cold, and *yin*, which is hot (hot and cold do not refer to temperature); hot conditions are treated with cold foods and treatments; cold conditions are treated with hot foods and treatments	Traditional healers	• Imbalance between the positive (yang) energy and the negative (yin) energy that are found in the body • Overexertion	Herbs, hot foods for conditions associated with yin conditions and cold foods for conditions associated with yang conditions; home remedies and folk medicines
Hispanic Americans	Body contains four humors (fluids) that need to be balanced. Illness develops from imbalance. Humors are blood (hot, moist); phlegm (cold, moist); black bile (cold, dry); yellow bile (hot, dry)	Native healers (Jerbero, Curandera)	• Punishment from God for sins	Candles, prayers, wearing medals, hot and cold foods to restore balance of humors

Native Americans	Spiritual powers control body's energy; harmony must exist between body, mind, and spirit; illness results when harmony is disrupted	• Violation of taboo • Attack by witch or evil spirits • Do not believe in germ theory	Medicine man, shaman	Sand painting to diagnose condition and determine treatment; elaborate rituals; carrying medicine bundles; wearing masks to hide from or frighten evil spirits
African Americans	Body, mind, and spirit must be in harmony for health; life is a process rather than a state; illness can occur if self-care is not taken	• Punishment from God • Spirits and demons	Folk practitioners, root workers	Prayer, diet, home remedies, wearing copper and silver bracelets, wearing talismans and amulets
Islamic Americans	Magico-religious: emotional distress; expressed as "heart disease"; feel responsible to visit and help ill; the individual has no control over life events, as good and evil usually are result of "will of Allah"; male-dominated society with male children more highly valued than female children; may use female circumcision to ensure faithfulness and be accepted by the women; may resist medical direction	Will of Allah; punishment for sins; various beliefs in causes such as imbalance of hot and cold; influence of an "Evil Eye"	Traditional healers; physicians	Magico-religious; prayer; self-care and medical science; use amulets inscribed with verses from the Koran; turquoise stones; charm of a hand with five fingers to protect against the evil eye; male health professionals prohibited from touching or examining females; males may refuse health care from females

169

- Some patients may wear garments, jewelry, or cover certain areas of the body because of religious practices.
- Some patients will have specific rituals for washing, peri care, and personal hygiene.

RELIGIOUS BELIEFS

You can support your patient's spirituality and religious practices by:
- Being a willing listener
- Respecting the patient's belief system
- Never trying to convert the patient to your belief system
- Respecting religious symbols
- Not interrupting during religious rites
- Reading aloud the patient's favorite passages from religious books such as the Bible, Talmud, Koran, or Book of Mormon
- Providing privacy during prayers and meditation or when clergy visits

Refer to Table 25-3.

CULTURAL SENSITIVITY

Guidelines for Developing Cultural Sensitivity
- Review your own belief systems.
- Consider how your own culture influences your behavior.
- Always view patients as individuals within a culture.
- Recognize that patients are a combination of heritage, culture, and community.
- Understand that culture influences how people behave and interact with others.
- Remember that personal space needs, eye contact, and ways of communicating are often culturally related.
- Recognize that some cultures have beliefs about health, wellness, and illness that are different from your own.

Table 25-3   COMMON RELIGIOUS BELIEF SYSTEMS

RELIGION	BELIEF IN A DEITY	VALUE OF PRAYER	BELIEF IN HEREAFTER	SPECIAL PRACTICES OR SYMBOLS
Protestant	Yes	Important	Yes	Baptism, Holy Communion, cross, Bible
Roman Catholic	Yes	Important	Yes	Baptism, Holy Communion, anointing the sick, reconciliation, Bible, medals, pictures, and statues of saints, rosaries, crucifix
Orthodox Judaism	Yes	Important	Yes	Torah, yarmulke (cap), tallith, menorah
Hinduism	Yes (many forms)	Important	Yes	No sacraments
Buddhism	Yes	Important	Yes	No sacraments
Muslims (Islam)	Yes	Important	Yes	Koran, prayer rug

There are individual variations in the belief and extent of practice.

- Be willing to modify care in keeping with the patient's cultural background and practices.
- Do not expect members of a cultural group to behave in exactly the same manner.
- Remember that patients' cultural values are deeply ingrained and not easily changed.
- Check with the nurse to learn special ways to deal with patients of different cultural backgrounds.
- Care for religious articles with respect.

- Provide privacy when a spiritual adviser is visiting the patient or the patient is practicing a devotional act.
- Try to learn about the practices, beliefs, and cultural heritage of the people who are most likely to be your patients. A library and the Internet are good sources.
- Ask patients politely about practices that are unfamiliar.
- Attend staff development classes designed to promote cultural sensitivity.

ENVIRONMENTAL AND NURSING ASSISTANT SAFETY

CHAPTER 26

THE PATIENT ENVIRONMENT

Hospital Beds

- The bed can be raised to the high horizontal position so there is less strain when giving care.
- The bed must be adjusted to the lowest horizontal position when you leave the room.
- Wheels should always be locked unless the bed is being moved.
- Review the nursing assistant safety information for using low beds in Chapter 30 of your book.

Side Rails

Benefits:
- Provide support and a "handle" for the patient to use for turning and repositioning in bed.
- Provide a "handle" for getting into and out of bed.
- Give the patient a feeling of security.
- Reduce the risk of falling out of bed when the patient is being transported from one location to another in bed.
- Provide access to bed and television controls that are part of the bed rail design.

Potential risks:
- Strangulation, suffocation, bodily injury, or death when the patient or part of the patient's body becomes entrapped between the bars of the side rails or between the side rails and the mattress.
- Serious injuries if the patient climbs over the rails and falls from this height.
- Skin tears, bruises, cuts, and scrapes.
- Agitation, caused by the feeling of being trapped or caged in.
- Feelings of isolation or restriction.
- Sadness because of loss of independence, having to call for help.
- Actual loss of independence, such as the ability to get up to use the bathroom or to retrieve an item dropped on the floor.

When side rails are used:
- They should be checked and attached securely before you leave the bedside unless ordered otherwise.
- They should be down only when the bed is in the lowest horizontal position.
- They should never be used for the attachment of tubes such as IV lines or catheters. Raising and lowering the side rails could put undue stress on such tubes and even pull them out.
- They should never be used for the attachment of restraints.
- Reassure the patient that raising the rails is hospital policy or a reminder of a new environment.
- Make sure the space between the mattress and side rails is not so large that it can cause entrapment.

INCIDENTS

When an accident occurs in the health care facility, it is referred to as an incident. An incident is any unexpected occurrence or event that interrupts normal procedures or causes a crisis. Incidents can cause harm to a patient, employee, or any other person. If you see an incident or are involved in one, you need to report it to your charge nurse.

Prevention of incidents depends on employees:

- Knowing their jobs and following all policies and procedures related to safety
- Maintaining a safe environment
- Knowing the patients and implementing safety measures to decrease their risk of injury

FIRE SAFETY

It is the responsibility of every staff member to know and regularly practice the fire and evacuation plans for the facility.

Fire Hazards

Some possible fire hazards include:

- Frayed electrical wires.
- Overloaded circuits.
- Plugs that are not properly grounded.
- Accumulated clutter such as papers and rags.
- Improper protection during oxygen therapy.
- Uncontrolled smoking; most health care facilities prohibit smoking throughout the facility.
- Matches left where children or others have unauthorized access to them.
- Smoking in rooms where oxygen is in use.

Other measures to reduce the risk of fires:

- Report smoke and/or burning smells.
- Keep all fire exits clear of equipment and debris.
- Know and practice fire drill safety.
- Do not let visitors give cigarettes to patients.
- Never permit smoking in bed.
- Some patients may need direct supervision when they smoke.
- Knowing and adhering to designated smoking areas, if any. Direct patients and visitors to the proper smoking areas. Most facilities prohibit smoking inside the building. Some do not permit smoking anywhere on the premises.

OXYGEN

When oxygen is in use:

- Never permit smoking, lighted matches, or open flames in the area.
- Do not use flammable liquids such as oils, alcohol, nail polish, aftershave, or perfume.
- Do not use electrical equipment such as radios, hair dryers, electric razors, heating pads, or toys.
- Post a sign indicating that oxygen is in use.
- Use cotton blankets and gowns for the patient.
- Wear cotton uniforms and non-wool sweaters when providing care.
- Be certain there are no cigarettes, matches, or lighters in the room.
- Do not adjust the liter flow.

IN CASE OF FIRE

In a fire emergency, remember RACE as defined here (Figure 26-1).

- R = Remove patients. Move patients to safety. Patients who can walk can be escorted. In some

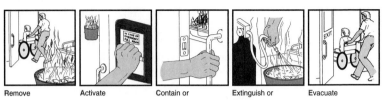

Remove   Activate   Contain or   Extinguish or   Evacuate

Figure 26-1 Sequence of critical actions in a fire.

cases, they may be called upon to assist others to escape routes. Patients may need to be moved in their beds out of the danger areas. If a person is unable to walk and the bed cannot be moved, bedsheets may be used as cradles and the patient pulled to safety.

- A = Activate (sound) the alarm. Use the intercom, emergency signal bell, telephone, or fire alarm as directed by facility policy. Give the location and type of fire.
- C = Contain fire. Close windows and doors to prevent drafts, which cause the fire to spread more rapidly.
- E = Extinguish fire or evacuate the area.

Use of a Fire Extinguisher

- Fire extinguishers should be carried upright.
- Remove the safety pin.
- Push the top handle down.
- Direct the hose nozzle at the base of the fire.

Remember the letters PASS:
P = PULL the pin.
A = AIM the nozzle at the base of the fire.
S = SQUEEZE the handle.
S = SWEEP back and forth along the base of the fire.

VIOLENCE IN THE WORKPLACE

Guidelines for Violence Prevention

- Follow all facility policies and procedures involving safety and security.
- Participate in continuing education programs to learn how to recognize and manage escalating agitation, assaultive behavior, or criminal intent.
- Attend classes on cultural diversity that offer sensitivity training on racial and ethnic issues and differences.
- If you are responsible for a secured area, control access to the area and keep it locked. Avoid propping open locked doors and windows. Never disable a door alarm.
- Do not leave keys unattended. Never share security alarm codes with unauthorized persons.
- Close shades or curtains at night.
- Report assaults or threats of assaults to the nurse manager immediately.
- Avoid wearing scarves, necklaces, earrings, and other jewelry that could cause injury to yourself if a patient or other individual attacks you.
- Do not carry valuables or large sums of cash to work.
- Avoid remote, dark areas when you are alone.

- Report lights that are burned out and locks that are not working.
- Exercise caution in elevators, stairwells, and unfamiliar areas. Immediately leave the area if you believe a hazard exists.
- Use the "buddy system" if personal safety may be threatened.
- If a patient or other person is "acting out," or you believe you may be assaulted, do not let the person come between you and the exit.
- Keep your head up, look ahead, and be aware of your surroundings.
- If your facility has security personnel, request that they escort you in dark or potentially dangerous areas. If no security personnel are on duty, ask other staff members to accompany you.
- Park in well-lighted areas. Always lock your car when parking. Look in the car before getting in, then lock the doors. Do not roll windows down to speak with individuals approaching your car.
- Report suspicious individuals or other potential safety hazards to the proper person. Never approach a suspicious person by yourself.

General Guidelines for Dealing with a Violent Individual

- Remain calm and avoid raising your voice, which may further agitate the perpetrator.
- Speak slowly, softly, and clearly.
- Call for help, if possible, or send someone to get help.
- Move away from heavy or sharp objects that may be used as weapons.
- Monitor your body language and avoid movements that could be challenging, such as placing your hands on your hips, moving toward the perpetrator, or pointing your finger or staring directly at the person. However, focus your attention on the person so you know what he or she is doing at all times.
- Position yourself at right angles to the perpetrator. Avoid standing directly in front of him or her. Maintain a distance of 3 to 6 feet.
- Position yourself so that an exit is accessible. Never let the perpetrator come between you and the exit.
- Avoid making sudden movements.
- Listen to what the person is saying. Encourage the person to talk. Communicate that you care and will genuinely try to help. Acknowledge that you understand he or she is upset. Break big problems into smaller, manageable ones.
- Avoid arguing and defensive statements. Accept criticism in a positive way. If you sincerely feel criticism is unwarranted, ask clarifying questions.
- Ask the person to leave and return when more calm.
- Ask questions to help regain control of the conversation.
- Avoid challenging, bargaining, or making promises you cannot keep.
- Describe the consequences of abusive behavior.
- Avoid touching an angry person.
- If a weapon is involved, ask the person to place it in a neutral location while you continue talking. Avoid trying to disarm the person, which may put you in danger.

ERGONOMICS

- Use correct body mechanics at all times, both at work and when you are off duty.
- Raise beds to a comfortable working height (remember to lower the beds when you finish your task).

- Use mechanical lifts when you need to transfer very heavy and/or dependent patients from the bed or chair and back.
- Use back supports if your employer requires them or if this is your preference. The use of back supports is controversial, but many nursing assistants find them helpful.

- Get another person to help when you need to transfer a patient who cannot bear his or her own weight fully.
- Use a cart to move heavy items.

Refer to Figures 26-2 and 26-3.

THE EIGHT COMMANDMENTS FOR LIFTING

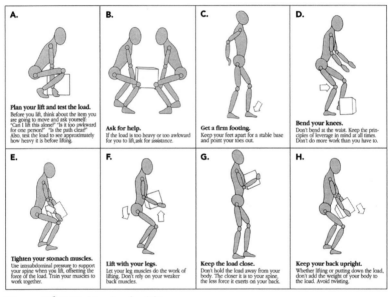

A.
Plan your lift and test the load.
Before you lift, think about the item you are going to move and ask yourself: "Can I lift this alone?" "Is it too awkward for one person?" "Is the path clear?" Also, test the load to see approximately how heavy it is before lifting.

B.
Ask for help.
If the load is too heavy or too awkward for you to lift, ask for assistance.

C.
Get a firm footing.
Keep your feet apart for a stable base and point your toes out.

D.
Bend your knees.
Don't bend at the waist. Keep the principles of leverage in mind at all times. Don't do more work than you have to.

E.
Tighten your stomach muscles.
Use intraabdominal pressure to support your spine when you lift, offsetting the force of the load. Train your muscles to work together.

F.
Lift with your legs.
Let your leg muscles do the work of lifting. Don't rely on your weaker back muscles.

G.
Keep the load close.
Don't hold the load away from your body. The closer it is to your spine, the less force it exerts on your back.

H.
Keep your back upright.
Whether lifting or putting down the load, don't add the weight of your body to the load. Avoid twisting.

Figure 26-2 Eight rules for lifting.

WARMING-UP EXERCISES TO PREVENT INJURIES

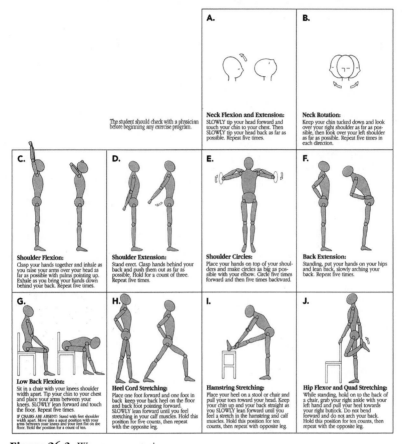

A.

Neck Flexion and Extension:
SLOWLY tip your head forward and touch your chin to your chest. Then SLOWLY tip your head back as far as possible. Repeat five times.

B.

Neck Rotation:
Keep your chin tucked down and look over your right shoulder as far as possible, then look over your left shoulder as far as possible. Repeat five times in each direction.

The student should check with a physician before beginning any exercise program.

C.

Shoulder Flexion:
Clasp your hands together and inhale as you raise your arms over your head as far as possible with palms pointing up. Exhale as you bring your hands down behind your back. Repeat five times.

D.

Shoulder Extension:
Stand erect. Clasp hands behind your back and push them out as far as possible. Hold for a count of three. Repeat five times.

E.

Shoulder Circles:
Place your hands on top of your shoulders and make circles as big as possible with your elbow. Circle five times forward and then five times backward.

F.

Back Extension:
Standing, put your hands on your hips and lean back, slowly arching your back. Repeat five times.

G.

Low Back Flexion:
Sit in a chair with your knees shoulder width apart. Tip your chin to your chest and place your arms between your knees. SLOWLY lean forward and touch the floor. Repeat five times.
IF CHAIRS ARE ABSENT: Stand with feet shoulder width apart. Move into a squat position with your arms between your knees and your feet flat on the floor. Hold the position for a count of ten.

H.

Heel Cord Stretching:
Place one foot forward and one foot in back keep your back heel on the floor and back foot pointing forward. SLOWLY lean forward until you feel stretching in your calf muscles. Hold this position for five counts, then repeat with the opposite leg.

I.

Hamstring Stretching:
Place your heel on a stool or chair and pull your toes toward your head. Keep your chin up and your back straight as you SLOWLY lean forward until you feel a stretch in the hamstring and calf muscles. Hold this position for ten counts, then repeat with opposite leg.

J.

Hip Flexor and Quad Stretching:
While standing, hold on to the back of a chair, grab your right ankle with your left hand and pull your heel towards your right buttock. Do not bend forward and do not arch your back. Hold this position for ten counts, then repeat with the opposite leg.

Figure 26-3 Warm-up exercises.

THE PATIENT'S MOBILITY: TRANSFER SKILLS

27

GUIDELINES FOR SAFE PATIENT TRANSFERS

Moving dependent patients can result in injury to you or the patient unless all safety measures are followed.

- Know the method of transfer that has been ordered by the nurse or physical therapist.
- Know the patient's capabilities.
- Use correct body mechanics.
- Place the bed in the lowest position before starting the standing transfer. Make sure the wheels on the bed and the transfer vehicle (wheelchair, stretcher) are locked before the move. It is helpful to elevate the head of the bed for a bed to chair transfer.
- *Never allow patients to place their hands on your body during a transfer.* This is a dangerous practice. A patient who is disoriented or frightened can cause you to lose your balance. If this happens, the patient can pull you down, possibly injuring both of you.
- *Never place your hands under a patient's arms or shoulders.* This practice can cause the patient severe shoulder injury.
- Use a transfer belt for standing transfers unless it is contraindicated.
- Make sure the patient is wearing shoes that are appropriate to the floor surface, and that clothing is not too loose or dragging on the floor.
- Be aware of any tubes, orthoses, or other items that must be dealt with during the transfer.
- Transfer the patient toward his or her strongest side if possible.
- Always explain to the patient what you are doing and how he or she can help.
- Allow the patient to see the surface to which he or she is being transferred. Encourage the patient to keep the head up.
- Stand close to the patient during the transfer.
- If the patient has a weak or paralyzed leg, brace the knee of that leg with your knee or leg. If the patient has a paralyzed arm, be sure it is supported during the transfer to avoid dangling and pulling on the patient's shoulder.
- Give the patient only the assistance that he or she needs.
- Never have the patient use a footstool unless it is absolutely necessary.
- Test the patient's understanding and make sure he or she knows what you expect of him or her during the transfer.
- Use an assistive device whenever possible.
- Know your limits.
- Get assistance from another worker whenever possible.

SELECTION OF TRANSFER

The method of transfer you select will depend on:

1. The patient's physical condition. This takes into consideration:
   - Paralysis (inability to move) of any extremity.
   - Paresis (weakness of an extremity).
   - Absence of an extremity due to amputation.
   - Recent hip surgery.
2. The patient's strength, endurance, and balance. These abilities are affected by:
   - Respiratory disease.
   - Cardiac disease.
   - Neurological disease such as multiple sclerosis or a stroke.
   - The ability to stand on one or both legs. This is called weight-bearing. The physician may order the patient to be non-weight-bearing or only partial weight-bearing if, for example, the patient has had hip surgery. For a standing transfer, the patient must be able to stand and have at least partial weight-bearing on one leg.
3. The patient's mental condition. Can the patient understand and follow instructions?
4. The patient's size. For example, a very tall or large person who cannot bear full weight would need two assistants or a mechanical lift.

Transfer Belts

A transfer belt is an assistive and safety device used to transfer or ambulate patients who need help. When it is used to assist a patient with ambulation, it is called a gait belt. If the patient has no ability to bear weight, then another method should be used for transferring.

Contraindications (situations in which something is not indicated or is inappropriate) for use of the transfer belt include:

- Abdominal, back, or rib injuries, fractures, or recent surgery
- Abdominal pacemakers
- Newly implanted medication pumps in the abdomen
- Advanced heart or lung disease
- Abdominal aneurysms
- Pregnancy
- Colostomy
- Gastrostomy tube, or feeding tube

Mechanical Lift

The mechanical lift is used when the patient is heavy, unable to assist, or unbalanced, or has an amputation or other condition that makes transfer with the belt difficult or impossible. *For safety reasons, the hydraulic lift should be operated by two or more nursing assistants. Never attempt to operate it alone. Some electric and battery-operated lifts can be safely used by one person. Know and follow your facility policy for use of the mechanical lift.*

THE PATIENT'S MOBILITY: AMBULATION

The term ambulate means to walk. The term gait refers to the way in which a person walks.

GUIDELINES FOR SAFE AMBULATION

- Encourage independent patients to use the hand rail when walking.
- Always stand on the patient's affected side when walking with her.
- Always use a gait belt (transfer belt) if the patient needs assistance with ambulation. Grasp the belt in the back with an underhand grip. Place your other hand on the patient's shoulder if balance is unsteady.
- Make sure the patient is wearing sturdy shoes with soles appropriate to the floor surface, and that laces are tied. Clothing should not be too loose or drag on the floor.
- Check floor for clutter or puddles that could cause a fall.
- If you are unsure of the patient's endurance or balance, ask another nursing assistant to follow behind you with a wheelchair. If the patient becomes weak, dizzy, or tired, she can sit in the wheelchair.
- Check rubber tips on bottoms of canes, crutches, and walkers and the rubber handgrips. These should be replaced if the ridges are cracked, loose, or worn down. If the ridges are filled with debris, use alcohol and cotton swabs to clean them. Replace the handgrip if it is loose or cracked.
- Check screws, nuts, and bolts for tightness. Do not use any device that appears unsafe. Report the problem to the appropriate person.
- Practice good body mechanics for both yourself and the patient.
- Teach the patient to practice safety.
- Position your body so it moves with the patient's body. You should not interfere with the patient's movement. Match the patient's stride.
- Encourage the patient to stand upright and erect when walking.
- Encourage the patient to take large, even steps. Teach him or her to maintain a wide base of support. The distance between the feet should be equal to the patient's shoulder width.
- Allow adequate time for ambulation. Avoid making the patient feel rushed.
- Allow the patient time to rest, if necessary.
- Provide only the amount of assistance necessary.
- If the patient is not motivated, place a chair ahead of him or her. Tell the patient the goal is to walk to the chair.
- Stop ambulation immediately if the patient shows signs of illness, pain, extreme fatigue, shortness of breath, dizziness, sweating, or anxiety. Notify the nurse.
- Never leave the patient standing unattended. When you are through, leave the patient safely sitting in a chair.

THE FALLING PATIENT

If a patient starts to fall, you must protect both yourself and the patient.

- Do not try to hold him or her upright.
- Ease the patient to the floor, letting him or her slide down your bended knee.
- Call the nurse to assess the patient for injuries before he or she is moved.

If you find a patient on the floor:

- Remain in the room and call for help.
- Leave the patient on the floor.
- Provide emergency measures that you are qualified to provide.

USE OF WHEELCHAIRS

A wheelchair enables a patient to gain independence. The wheelchair should fit the person using it. Correct fit and body alignment will prevent contractures. If the chair fits correctly, there will be:

- About 4 inches between the top of the back upholstery and the patient's axillae.
- Armrests that support the arms without pushing the shoulders up or forcing them to hang.
- Two to 3 inches clearance between the front edge of the seat and the back of the patient's knee.
- Enough space between the patient's hip and the chair to slide your hand between the patient's hips on each side and the side of the wheelchair; the right amount of space prevents internal or external rotation of the hips.
- Two inches between the bottom of the footrests and the floor.
- 90-degree angles between the feet and the legs, whether they are on the footrests or on the floor (when the footrests have been removed).

- Review the information on proper chair and wheelchair positioning in Chapter 8 of your book.

If the wheelchair does not fit the patient, obtain another chair, or check with the nurse or physical therapist to see how you can use pads or other devices to adapt the chair to the patient.

Guidelines for Wheelchair Safety

- Check wheelchairs to see that brakes are working and wheels are securely attached. If the patient needs footrests, make sure they are in place. Replace arm of wheelchair if it was removed during transfer.
- The small, front caster wheels of the chair provide the ability to move in all directions. The large part of the wheel faces back when the chair is moving. When the chair is parked, position the large part of the front wheel facing forward. This changes the center of gravity in the chair. Positioning the wheels to face forward prevents tipping if the patient leans forward. It helps stabilize the chair if the patient picks up an item from the floor. To reposition the wheels, back the chair up, then move it forward.
- Keep the wheelchair locked when not moving.
- Apply brakes and lift footrests out of the way when the patient is getting in or out of the wheelchair.
- Instruct the patient not to try to pick up an object off the floor. If there is satisfactory trunk stability and balance, the patient may be taught to do so, but instruct the patient to:
  - Avoid shifting weight in the direction of the reach
  - Not move forward in the seat
  - Not reach down between the knees

The safest method is to position the chair alongside the object with casters in forward position, lock the chair, and reach only as far as the arm will extend.

- Check the patient's body alignment while in the wheelchair and reposition the patient when necessary.
- Prevent bath blankets, lap robes, or clothing from getting caught in wheels.
- Observe the patient's affected arm. A paralyzed arm may fall over the side of the wheelchair and become caught in the wheel.
- Guide the wheelchair from behind, grasping both handgrips.
- Approach corners slowly and look before you go around them.
- Take care when approaching swinging doors. Prop the door open to propel the chair through the door. If this is not possible, back through swinging doors.
- Back the wheelchair over the threshold in a doorway or elevator.
- When leaving the elevator, push the stop button and ask others to step out. Turn the wheelchair around and back it out the door.
- When transporting a patient in a wheelchair down a ramp or incline, walk backward, slowly pulling the chair. Periodically look over your shoulder, as you would when backing up in a car to make sure that the path is clear.
- When parking a wheelchair, avoid blocking a doorway. Apply the brakes.

Positioning the Dependent Patient in a Wheelchair

The dependent patient may slide down in the wheelchair, requiring assistance to regain body alignment. Several procedures can be used to correct the dependent patient's position in the wheelchair. Lock the drive wheels and position the caster wheels in the forward position before repositioning the patient.

1. Stand in front of the patient; make sure that the feet are in alignment and the arms are on the armrests. Help the patient lean forward and push with the hands and legs as you push against the patient's knees.

2. For an alternate method, place a soft towel or small sheet under the patient's buttocks and use this as a pull sheet to move the patient up in the chair. This requires two people. Devices such as the TLC pad (Figure 28-1) enable one or two caregivers to safely pull the patient back or reposition in the wheelchair.

3. This method also requires two people. Place the transfer belt around the patient's waist. One assistant stands in back of the wheelchair and grasps the transfer belt with one hand on each side of the patient. The other one stands in front of the patient and places his or her hands and arms under the patient's knees. On the count of three, this assistant supports the lower extremities while the other one moves the patient back in the chair. This method is not recommended for a heavy patient.

4. This method also requires two people. Stand in back of the wheelchair and have another assistant in front of the patient. Both assistants work with knees and hips bent and backs straight. Lean forward with your head over the patient's shoulder. Instruct the patient to fold the arms. Place your arms around the patient's trunk. Grasp the patient's right wrist with your left hand and his or her left wrist with your right

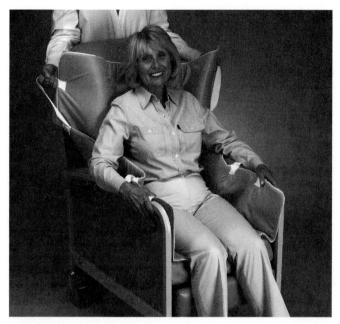

Figure 28-1 The TLC pad may be used by one or two nursing assistants to move the patient back and up in a chair. It is also used for bed positioning and for moving patients from the floor to bed. (Courtesy of Skil-Care Corporation, Yonkers, NY, (800) 431-2972.)

hand. The other assistant encircles the patient's knees with hands and arms. On the count of three, both assistants lift and move the patient up.

5. One person can perform this procedure. The patient needs to be oriented and able to follow directions. Stand in front of the patient. Flex your knees and hips and keep your back straight. Position your feet, one on each side of the patient's feet. Brace your knees against the patient's knees. Have the patient lean forward. Lean forward over the patient's right shoulder, with the patient's head under your right arm. Encircle your arms around the patient's trunk. The patient's arms are folded together. Rock the patient forward, and on

the count of three, when his or her weight is over the legs, push against the patient's knees to move back in the chair.

If the patient can bear weight, it is easier and more beneficial to assist him or her to stand and then sit back down, getting the hips to the back of the chair. Wedge cushions placed in the wheelchair will prevent the patient from sliding forward. However, if forward sliding is an ongoing problem for a patient, make sure the wheelchair "fits" the patient correctly. (An improperly fitted chair is a common cause of forward sliding.) A seat that is too long shifts the patient's weight to the sacrum and coccyx, making it much more difficult to propel the chair. It also increases discomfort, pressure, and the risk of skin breakdown. Some patients slide forward, closer to the front edge of the chair to compensate for the seat length. Some appear as if they will fall on the floor, so staff may consider restraints or alternatives to keep the person in the chair. Obtaining a chair that fits is easier and better for the patient. When the patient is seated properly, the hips should be near the back of the seat. The front edge of the seat should end two or three inches before the back of the patient's knees. Remember that good positioning always begins with the feet: Be sure the patient's feet are well supported on the footrests or floor. The knees should not be higher than the hips.

Wheelchair Activity

Pressure over the buttocks is dramatically increased when the patient is sitting. Teach the patient (and provide assistance if necessary) to periodically relieve the pressure by shifting weight every 15 minutes. *Be sure the wheelchair is locked before beginning any activities involving the patient's movement in the chair.*

Wheelchair Push-Ups

1. Teach the patient to place one hand on each armrest, keeping both elbows bent.
2. Then have the patient lean forward slightly, pushing on the armrests and straightening the elbows while lifting the buttocks off the seat of the wheelchair. Have the patient hold this position to the count of five if possible.

Leaning

If the patient cannot do push-ups, teach him or her to place the hands on the armrests or thighs and lean forward slightly, and then to each side to relieve pressure on the buttocks. Monitor

patients with balance problems to avoid their falling out of the chair.

TRANSPORTING A PATIENT BY STRETCHER

- Before moving a patient on a stretcher, make sure that the side rails are up and all safety belts are fastened.
- Push the stretcher by standing at the patient's head. Moving the stretcher in this manner enables you to use good body mechanics and to see potential hazards.
- Approach corners slowly and look before you go around them.
- Take care when approaching swinging doors. Prop the door open to propel the stretcher through the door. If this is not possible, back through swinging doors.
- When entering an elevator, push the stop button to lock the doors open. Back the stretcher into the elevator by walking backward and pulling the head end. Stand by the patient's head while the elevator is in motion. When the elevator stops, push the stop button to lock the door open. Push the stretcher out so the feet exit the elevator first. If the threshold is uneven, go to the foot end of the stretcher and pull it out of the elevator. After the stretcher is safely out of the elevator, unlock the door mechanism.
- When transporting a stretcher down a ramp or incline, walk backward, slowly guiding the stretcher from the head end. Periodically look over your shoulder to make sure that the path is clear.
- When parking a stretcher, avoid blocking a doorway. Never leave a patient unattended and unsupervised on a stretcher.

ADMISSION, TRANSFER, AND DISCHARGE

ADMISSION

- Prepare the room and any special equipment.
- Introduce yourself and observe the patient carefully.
- Listen for complaints as you escort and assist the patient to the room and to bed.
- Initial observations are very important. They become the basis of comparison for future observations.
- Make sure the patient knows how to use the call signal before you leave the room.

If it is necessary to ask visitors to leave, do so in a kindly and polite manner. They will be most anxious to remain and see the patient settled and comfortable, so:

- Show them where they may wait.
- Let them know about how long they will have to wait.
- Tell them where they can get refreshments.
- Answer questions they may have about where to find a chapel and telephones, and about visiting hours.
- After you have completed your part of the admission procedure, locate visitors and let them know they may return to the patient's room.
- The patient's perception of what is happening may be affected by illness, pain, and fear. Making a good first impression on the patient and family members is important. If the first impression of the nursing

assistant is negative, this affects the patient's impression of all health care workers, and even the hospital. Do your best to provide a positive, professional impression.

FAMILY DYNAMICS

Family members are extensions of patients, and they usually must make adjustments when a loved one is admitted to the hospital. This is often an emotional time, with everyone in the family experiencing a spectrum of emotion ranging from relief at getting help to guilt because of the inability to care for the person at home. The family may also experience fear, anger, uncertainty, sadness, helplessness, and worry. Validate their feelings with comments such as, "I know this must be very difficult for you," as appropriate.

Understanding the emotions caused by facility admission will help you recognize why first impressions are important. Introduce yourself and explain your responsibilities as a nursing assistant. Use good communication skills and show that you care. Greet each patient and family member with warmth, courtesy, kindness, and respect. Make them feel welcome, and show that you are sincerely interested in the patient's well-being. Admission to the hospital does not have to be a negative experience. A competent, caring, professional staff will calm patient and family fears and turn a potentially negative experience into a positive one.

Guidelines for Family Dynamics

- Get to know family members and greet them warmly when they visit.
- Wear a name badge. Introduce yourself by name and position.
- Build positive and trusting relationships with family members.
- Make time to talk to the family. Listen to what they say and respond appropriately. Tell them about the patient's activities, as appropriate.
- If the family has been caring for the patient at home, they often know what works best. Listen to their advice about patient care. Pass the information on to the nurse.
- Show your appreciation, respect, and support of family caregivers.
- Inform the family about facility routines and services.
- Refer questions of a medical or personal nature to the nurse.
- Tactfully listen to suggestions, complaints, and comments. Inform the nurse, as appropriate.
- Inform the nurse if a visitor is upsetting a patient.
- Avoid judging family decisions. Remain neutral and stay out of family disagreements.
- Avoid gossiping with the family, and never discuss facility business with family members.
- Allow the family to participate in the patient's care, if the patient does not object. However, you should avoid making the family feel as if they are required to care for the patient. Avoid giving the impression that you are too busy to provide care.

TRANSFER

The patient may or may not fully understand the reasons for the transfer.

- Be positive and supportive in your attitude.

- Recognize that the patient may be feeling very anxious.

After the new unit has been notified and prepared for the move, you will:

- Tell the patient what you are doing.
- Gather all the patient's belongings together. Explain to the patient what you are doing.
- Get the patient's medicines, charts, and other personal data from the nurse.
- Assist in the physical transfer.
- Give the records and medication directly to the nurse on the new unit.

Caution: Never leave the patient, the records, or medications unattended.

- Make sure the patient is safe and comfortable in the new environment before you return to your own unit.

DISCHARGE PROCESS

The discharge, or authorized release, of a patient requires a written order from the physician. If a patient indicates an intention of leaving without an order, report it to the nurse immediately.

The patient should be spared any fatigue or unnecessary delay when being routinely discharged.

You can help if you:

- Check with the nurse to make sure that the physician has written an order for discharge before preparing the patient.
- Gather all the patient's belongings and assist in packing, if necessary.
- Carefully check the closet and bedside table. Disposable equipment is often sent home with the patient. If this is the policy in your facility, be sure that the equipment is clean.

- Check with the nurse for any medications or other treatment-related equipment that should be sent home with the patient.
- Verify that the patient has received discharge instructions from the nurse, physician, or discharge coordinator.
- Never allow a patient to leave the health care facility unassisted. The patient is the staff's responsibility until he or she has left the building.

BEDMAKING

Correct operation of any bed or equipment is important for patient safety. Always seek help and instruction from the nurse or another health care professional when using any specialized beds. Never try to operate any bed or equipment with a patient in it without first practicing and gaining security and skill in the procedures.

GUIDELINES FOR HANDLING LINENS AND MAKING THE BED

Handling Linens

1. Wash hands and use gloves if necessary; other personal protective equipment may be required.
2. Laundry hampers placed in the hallway should be at least one room away from clean linen carts or according to facility policy.
3. The clean linen cart is always covered; put the covers back in place after removing required linen.
4. Take only the linens you need into the patient's room.
5. Linens that touch the floor are considered dirty and are placed in the laundry hamper; they are not used.
6. Avoid contact between the linens and your uniform (for both clean and soiled linens).
7. Unused linen is never returned to the clean linen cart; it is placed in the laundry hamper.

8. As soiled linen is removed from the bed, keep the soiled areas on the inside and fold or roll the linen toward the center.
9. Never shake bed linens, because microbes will be released into the air.
10. Soiled linen is never placed on environmental surfaces in the room, such as overbed table, chair, or floor; soiled linens are placed in the appropriate laundry hamper (follow facility policy).
11. Fill laundry hampers no more than two-thirds full. Keep the lid to the hamper on tightly at all times.
12. Many facilities do not permit laundry hampers or barrels to be taken into the patient's room. Soiled linen may be placed in a plastic bag or a pillowcase in the room. Make a cuff at the top of the bag or open end of the pillowcase and place the cuff over the back of the chair. When the bag or case is two-thirds full, secure the top and place it in the hamper in the hallway.
13. Laundry hampers or barrels are returned to the utility room after use, or as directed by facility policy.
14. Remember the chain of infection. To prevent infection, wash your hands before handling clean linen. Wear gloves to remove soiled linen contaminated (or potentially contaminated) with bloodborne pathogens, secretions, and excretions.

15. Discard your soiled gloves in a plastic bag or covered container. Avoid environmental contamination with used gloves. Wash your hands at the sink or use alcohol-based hand cleaner after removing gloves and before placing clean linen on the bed. Never make the bed while wearing soiled gloves. No gloves are necessary in most unoccupied bedmaking situations. If gloves are needed for the occupied bedmaking procedure, discard soiled gloves after removing soiled linen. Wash your hands. Apply clean gloves before continuing.

Making the Bed

1. Use proper body mechanics at all times to prevent back injury.
2. Work on one side of the bed at a time to complete removal of soiled linen and placement of clean linen.
3. Make sure the bottom sheet and draw sheet (if used) are smooth and unwrinkled (wrinkles in bed linens can lead to skin breakdown, especially for patients who must remain in bed).
4. Follow the care plan for positioning the head and foot of the bed, the number of pillows to be used, and the use of pillows for positioning.

Bed linen is always changed when soiled. It is routinely changed:
- Daily in the acute care facility
- Two or three times a week in long-term care facilities

LOW BEDS

Studies suggest that up to 54% of all falls from bed occur over the elevated siderails. Low beds reduce the risk of falling from a great height. They are usually used without bed rails. Adult patients who are at risk for falling from bed are usually good candidates for low bed use. However, patients who have had hip replacement surgery within the previous 90 days should not use low beds.

Low beds are wonderful tools for reducing injuries related to patient falls, but having one or more low beds on the unit increases the risk for staff injuries. Nursing assistants must have good organizational skills and use common sense when preparing to work with the patient in or make the low bed. Using good body mechanics is essential when lifting, moving, and caring for patients, and making beds.

Guidelines for Caring for Patients in Low Beds

- For maximum safety, place the far side of the bed against a wall.
- Move other furnishings far enough away from the bed to prevent injury.
- Keep the bed in the lowest horizontal position with the wheels locked when the patient is in bed.
- If the bed you are using has a high-low feature, use it whenever caring for the bedfast patient, transferring the patient, and making the bed.
- Place a high-impact, padded, plastic-covered mat on the floor next to the low bed to protect and cushion the patient in the event of a fall.
- Although a floor pad or mat reduces the risk of patient injury from falls, it presents a trip hazard for staff.
  - Fold and store the mat when the patient is out of bed.
  - Move slowly and carefully when working near a floor mat.
  - Avoid entering the room in total darkness. Leave a night light on, or turn the light on when entering.

- Avoid leaning forward or down at the waist to provide patient care. Elevate the height of the bed, sit in a chair, squat, kneel on one or both knees, or sit on the mat, depending on the nature of your activity at the bedside.
- Elevate the bed to the proper height for the patient when transferring him or her out of bed. A one quarter size side rail or pole that extends from floor to ceiling is helpful for the patient to grasp when getting into or out of bed.
  - Discourage the patient from grabbing items such as the overbed table, chair, or sink.
- Use good body mechanics, a transfer belt, and a ceiling or mechanical lift when assisting patients into and out of bed.
- Follow the instructions on the care plan.
- Evaluate the overall safety of the room and bed. Remove trip and fall hazards and other items that may cause injury.

Guidelines for Making Low Beds

When making a low bed, modify the regular bedmaking procedure by using these adaptations to reduce your risk of injury. You should:

- Plan to make low beds with a partner, if possible.
- Mentally plan and prepare yourself for the procedure.
- Gather everything you will need before entering the room. Double-check to make sure you have all needed items.
- Think about what you are doing. Organize and plan your work to reduce the total number of motions needed to complete the task.

- Elevate the height of the bed, if possible.
- Place linen and needed items on the chair or other clean area within close reach of the bed.
- Avoid moving quickly. Rapid motion increases your risk of injury.
- Use good body mechanics, maintain a neutral posture and bend from the legs. Avoid bending at the waist or twisting.
- During the bedmaking procedure, you may squat, sit, or kneel (on one or both knees) on the plastic mat next to the bed if doing so is easier for you and helps keep your spine straight. Your position is somewhat determined by height: A tall person may be able to sit on the mat while making the bed, whereas a shorter person may need to squat.
- Never handle clean linen while wearing soiled gloves.
- Avoid environmental contamination with your used gloves.
- Check the bed for lost items, such as glasses, hearing aid, or dentures, and remove them if found.
- *Slowly* remove the bed linen *several pieces at a time*. Avoid rolling the linen up and trying to remove it all in one bundle.
  - The weight of the linen and your posture increase the risk of back injury.
  - Roll the used side of the linen inward and remove one or two pieces at a time.
- Place soiled linen in a plastic bag well to the side on the mat, in a pillowcase draped over the back of the chair, in a plastic bag on the seat of a second chair, or according to facility policy.
  - Despite your proximity to the floor, avoid placing clean or soiled linen on the floor.

- Do not change position or waste steps by removing linen from the room until you have finished the bedmaking procedure.
- Remove your gloves and discard in a second plastic bag or according to facility policy.
- After removing soiled linen, handwashing is necessary before handling clean linen. Do not be tempted to omit this important step.
- Carry a pocket-size bottle of alcohol-based hand cleaner. Do a 15-second handwash with the alcohol cleaner before handling clean linen.
- Make one side of the bed at a time. This is faster, more efficient, requires fewer physical motions, and conserves energy.
- Use a fitted bottom sheet to reduce the number of movements necessary for making the bed, thereby lowering the risk of back strain.
- If one side of the bed is next to the wall, leave the bed in the high position, if permitted by your facility. If the bed is not near a wall, raise the rail on the far side, or position it at the lowest horizontal height, or position according to facility policy.
- Wipe the mat with disinfectant, then fold and store it under the bed, or according to facility policy.
- Perform your procedure completion actions and remove and discard soiled linen, gloves, and other procedural trash when you leave the room. You may use alcohol hand cleaner during this step of the procedure, as well, unless your hands are visibly soiled.

PRINCIPLES OF NUTRITION AND FLUID BALANCE

POSTSURGERY DIET PROGRESSION

The progression of diets a patient is allowed following surgery is as follows:
1. Ice chips/sip of water
2. Clear liquids
3. Full liquids
4. Soft diet
5. Regular diet

TYPES OF DIETS

Liquid Diets

Clear Liquid Diet

A clear liquid diet is a temporary diet because it is inadequate for meeting nutritional needs. It is made up primarily of water and carbohydrates for energy and is intended to replace fluids that may have been lost through vomiting or diarrhea. Feedings are given every 2, 3, or 4 hours as prescribed by the physician. When a clear liquid food item is held up to the light, you can see through it. The clear liquid diet consists of liquids that do not irritate, cause gas formation, or encourage bowel movements (defecation).

Foods allowed on the clear diet include:
• Tea or coffee with sugar but without cream
• Strained fruit or vegetable juice with gelatin (occasionally)

• Fat-free meat broths
• Ginger ale (usually), other soda drinks, strained grape or apple juice
• Gelatin (occasionally)
• Popsicles

Full Liquid Diet

This diet does supply nourishment and may be used for longer periods of time than the clear liquid diet. Six to 8 ounces are usually given every 2 to 3 hours.

The full liquid diet is given to:
• Those with acute infections
• Patients who have difficulty chewing
• Those who have conditions that involve the digestive tract

The diet includes all the foods allowed on the clear liquid diet, as well as the following:
• Strained cereal (gruel)
• Strained soups
• Sherbet
• Gelatin
• Eggnog
• Malted milk
• Milk and cream
• Plain ice cream
• Strained vegetables and fruit juices
• Junket
• Solids that liquefy at room temperature
• Yogurt

Soft Diet

The soft diet usually follows the full liquid diet. Although this diet

nourishes the body, between-meal feedings are sometimes given to increase calorie count. Foods allowed on the soft diet are:
- Low-residue, which are almost completely used by the body
- Mildly flavored, slightly seasoned, or unseasoned
- Prepared in a form that requires little digestion

The diet includes liquids and semi-solid foods that have a soft texture and are easily digested. It is given to patients who:
- Have infections and fevers
- Have difficulty chewing
- Have conditions that involve the digestive tract
- Are on a progressive postoperative dietary regime

The following foods are usually allowed on the soft diet:
- Soups
- Cream cheese and cottage cheese
- Crackers, toast
- Fish
- White meat of chicken or turkey (boiled or stewed)
- Fruit juices
- Cooked fruit (sieved)
- Tea, coffee
- Milk, cream, butter
- Cooked cereals
- Eggs (not fried)
- Beef and lamb (scraped or finely ground)
- Cooked vegetables (mashed or sieved)
- Angel or sponge cake
- Small amounts of sugar
- Gelatin, custard
- Pudding
- Plain ice cream

Foods to be avoided include:
- Coarse cereals
- Spices
- Gas-forming foods (onions, cabbage, beans)
- Rich pastries and desserts
- Foods high in roughage/fiber
- Fried foods
- Raw fruits and vegetables
- Corn
- Pork (except crisp bacon)

Special Diets

Religious practice requires changes in diet for some patients. Some faith restrictions are summarized in Table 31-1.

Therapeutic Diets

Standard diets can be changed to conform to special dietary requirements. For example, an order might be written for a low-sodium soft diet when a patient has ill-fitting dentures and heart disease. Commonly prescribed therapeutic diets include the diabetic diet, sodium-restricted diet, and low-fat diet.

The Diabetic Diet

Diet is an integral part of the therapy of the patient with diabetes mellitus. The diet is nutritionally adequate. It provides enough energy in the form of calories for a 24-hour period. Sometimes a proper diet is all that is needed to control the disease. Usually, however, the food intake is balanced by the administration of insulin or hypoglycemic drugs.

It is important for you to accurately evaluate and report the patient's intake. Foods and liquids have a significant impact on diabetes management. Illness increases the need for insulin because the liver releases more glucose in response to stress. Dehydration is a particularly serious problem for the diabetic. This can occur when not enough foods and fluids are taken

Table 31-1 RELIGIOUS DIETARY PRACTICES

FAITH	COFFEE	TEA	ALCOHOL	PORK/PORK PRODUCTS	CAFFEINE-CONTAINING FOODS	DAIRY PRODUCTS	ALL MEATS
					(RESTRICTED FOOD)		
Christian Science	•	•	•				
Roman Catholic							1 hour before communion, Ash Wednesday, Good Friday
Latter-Day Saints (Mormons)	•	•	•		•		
Seventh-Day Adventist	•	•	•	•	•		Many are vegetarians, some well-cooked, lean meats permitted
Some Baptist	•	•	•				
Greek Orthodox (on fast days)						•	Fasting from meat and dairy products on Wed./Fri. during Lent and other holy days
Jewish Orthodox				• Also shellfish		Certain holy days	Forbids the serving of milk and milk products with meat; regulates food preparation; forbids cooking on the Sabbath
Muslim, Islamic			•	•			Fasting during Ramadan during day, feasting at night
Hindu							Some are vegetarians
Buddhist							Meat must be blessed and killed in special ways; some sects are vegetarians

in. Insulin administration may depend on your observations.

- Some physicians prescribe a very carefully balanced diet and insulin to maintain the level of blood sugar (glucose) within normal limits. All foods must be measured, and repeated injections of insulin are required.
- Other physicians are much more liberal in their approach. They permit an unmeasured diet, limiting only sugar and high-sugar foods. This diet is known as a no-concentrated-sweets diet. It may be balanced by insulin or hypoglycemic drugs.
- Many physicians treat diabetes with an approach that is midway between the preceding two methods. They prescribe diets with specific calorie levels, such as a 1,200-calorie diet or the 1,500-calorie diet. The diet is balanced by insulin or hypoglycemic drugs.

Sodium-Restricted Diet

Sodium-restricted diets may be ordered for patients with chronic renal failure and cardiovascular disease. Diets that are moderately, mildly, or severely restricted in sodium content may be prescribed. These diets are among the most difficult for patients to follow. Some foods have significant levels of sodium added during processing, and others naturally contain relatively large amounts of sodium. These foods may be restricted for a sodium-restricted diet. They include:

- Meat
- Fish
- Poultry
- Milk and milk products
- Eggs

  Avoid:
- Pork
- Potato chips

- Pop (soda) containing sodium
- Pickles
- Processed meats
- Canned foods, such as vegetables and soups

Some foods are naturally low in sodium and can be used more liberally. They are:

- Some cereals, such as shredded wheat
- Vegetables
- Fruits

Low-Fat/Low-Cholesterol Diet

Low-fat/low-cholesterol diets are prescribed for patients who suffer from vascular, heart, liver, or gallbladder disease and for those who have difficulty with fat metabolism. Fats are limited, and calories are balanced by increasing proteins and carbohydrates. Foods are baked, roasted, or broiled, and the skin is removed from chicken. Low-fat foods include:

- Low-fat cottage cheese (no other allowed)
- Skim milk, buttermilk, yogurt
- Lean meats, fish, chicken
- Vegetables and fruits
- Jams, jellies, ices
- Cereals, pasta, bread, potatoes, rice
- Carbonated beverages, tea, coffee

Mechanically Altered Diets

Any diet can be mechanically altered. This means that the consistency and texture are modified, making the food easier to chew and swallow. The mechanical soft diet is commonly served to patients with no teeth or to those with serious dental problems. Meats and hard foods are ground to the consistency of hamburger. Soft items, such as bread, are not ground. In the pureed diet, food is blended with gravy or liquid until it is the consistency of pudding. This diet is used for patients who have difficulty swallowing. Pureed foods should not be watery. Properly prepared food items will support a plastic spoon in the upright position.

Supplements, Nourishments, and Snacks

Nutritional supplements are dietary supplements given to patients for a specific therapeutic purpose. Supplements usually contain extra vitamins, minerals, and nutrients. Most are a source of extra calories, although some are low-calorie. They contain dietary ingredients that are essential to the patient's diet. They are often given to patients who have experienced weight loss and those who need additional calories to meet a medical need. Other special supplements are ordered by the physician or dietitian to treat patients with specific medical needs, such as those with renal failure, pressure ulcers, diabetes, chronic obstructive pulmonary disease, or HIV. In most facilities, the nursing assistant must document the percentage of the product the patient consumed on a flow sheet. Nutritional supplements:

- are ordered by the physician or dietitian.
- are given for a specific therapeutic purpose.
- are not nutritionally complete, and are not a replacement for meals.
- are given to make up for a nutritional deficiency, strengthen the patient, or promote healing.
- come in a variety of preparations and flavors to promote patient acceptance.
- usually taste best when served cold.
- contain approximately 250 calories per can, or about 1 calorie per mL.
- are usually lactose-free, and higher in sodium and protein than most tube feeding formulas.
- are flavored and are used for oral nutrition. They are not recommended for tube feedings, and tube feeding formulas are not recommended for nutritional supplementation. (Tube feeding formulas are not flavored.)
- usually taste good and are well accepted. Most patients believe they taste like a milkshake, although most are lactose-free and do not contain milk products.
- are very filling, and should *never be given* with meals or immediately before meal time.
- are expensive and should not be wasted!

Nourishments are substantial food items given to patients to increase nutrient intake. They are often planned and ordered by the facility dietitian and include foods such as:

- sandwiches
- instant breakfast
- milkshakes
- pudding
- whole or chocolate milk
- yogurt
- cottage cheese
- ice cream or sherbet
- liquid milk-type products, such as Great Shake® and Shake Up® are also used

Nourishments are usually given between meals to provide needed nutrients or prevent hunger. Serving snacks, nourishments, and supplements is an important nursing assistant responsibility.

Snacks may be planned and regularly given, or unplanned upon patient request. Regular food items are usually given as requested by the patient. No special order is needed. They are given to patients to prevent or eliminate hunger between meals.

To serve supplements and nourishments:

- Wash your hands.

- Check the nourishment list of each patient for any limitations or special dietary instructions.
- Allow patients to choose from the available nourishments whenever possible.
- Assist those who are unable to take their nourishment alone.
- Remember to pick up used glasses and dishes after the patient has finished and return them to the proper area.
- Notice what the patient was or was not able to take.
- Record on intake and output (I&O) sheet if required.

CALORIE COUNTS AND FOOD INTAKE STUDIES

The physician or dietitian may order special food intake studies for patients with special nutritional needs.

- The patient's food intake is carefully recorded for a period of time, usually 3 days.
- A special food documentation form is prepared and placed on the medical record or other designated location.
- The food intake study usually begins with the breakfast meal on the day after the physician writes the order.
- Some facilities post a sign in the room or on the door to remind staff and visitors that a study is in progress.
- At the end of each meal, you will carefully and accurately record the patient's food intake on the form.

FOOD THICKENERS

When adding thickeners:
- Use the correct product.
- Use the correct amount.
- Follow the manufacturer's directions.
- Stir the thickener well.

- Follow the speech therapist's instructions and plan of care for positioning and feeding.

HUMAN SENSORY RESPONSE TO FOOD

The human sensory response to food is complicated. The brain coordinates signals of smell and taste with sight, temperature, and texture. Sensory disorders have many causes, and are often difficult to overcome. Sensory problems may affect food:
- temperature
- smell
- taste
- hearing and vision
- touch
- texture

The presentation and attractiveness of food are especially important for patients whose smell, taste, texture, and temperature sensations are impaired. Always check food temperature. Patients are at risk of burns if food is too hot. Patients with abnormal temperature sensations are at greater risk than others. Some patients will be unable to smell the food. Taste and texture sensations may be altered, causing the food to taste unusual or be unappetizing to the patient. Tiny bumps on the tongue, called *papillae,* are usually called "taste buds." These are impaired in aging and some medical conditions. Humans have five known taste buds, but this is an area in which further study is needed. The taste buds that have been identified are:
- sweet
- salt
- bitter
- sour
- *umami*

Umami is a Japanese word for which there is no English equivalent. This taste bud was first identified as a taste bud in 2000. Umami is a savory, meaty, or protein taste, such as that of a good steak or sauteed mushrooms. Salt and some other substances are believed to amplify the response of the taste buds, probably by acting as an electrical conductor.

DOCUMENTING MEAL INTAKE

Each facility has a policy and procedure for documenting and recording the amount of food patients consume at each meal. Every staff member should use the same method of calculation and documentation. The system may also be used for snacks, nourishments, and supplements. A clipboard is commonly used to record meal intake. The clipboard is usually on top of the cart where used trays are returned. After the meal, the information is transferred to the patient's chart. Remember that documented information is confidential. Keep the information covered with a piece of paper when the clipboard is not in use. Examples of methods of documenting meal intake are pictured in Figures 31-1 and 31-2.

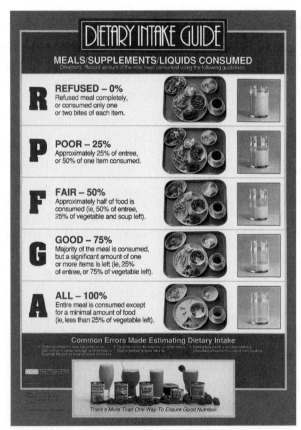

Figure 31-1 Accurate documentation of meal intake is an important nursing assistant responsibility. (Used with permission of Ross Products Division, Abbott Laboratories, Columbus, Ohio.)

A	
Alternate method of documenting meal intake	
Breakfast	
Egg, cheese, or cottage cheese	50%
Hot or cold cereal	30%
Bread	10%
Bacon, ham, or sausage	10%
Total	100%

Occasionally, a patient will request no protein foods (eggs, meat, cheese, cottage cheese) at breakfast. Please reassign the percentages to the other items on the tray and document accordingly.

Lunch and Supper	
Meat, egg, cheese, or cottage cheese	40%
Starchy vegetable	20%
Vegetable or salad	20%
Bread	10%
Dessert	10%
Total	100%

The meat and starchy vegetables may be combined in some dishes, such as casseroles. If so, add the point values for these items together to total 60%. Sandwiches are also 60% because the two bread slices are the starchy vegetable. An additional bread item such as crackers may also be served at the meal.

B

Alternate method of documenting meal intake

	Food Item	Percentage of Meal
Breakfast		
	eggs	35%
	eggs and bacon	40%
	eggs and sausage	45%
	toast *or* cereal	30%
	milk	20%
	fruit juice	15%
Dinner and Supper	meat group, including eggs, main dish, legumes	50%
	fruit group, including dessert items	15%
	bread or cereal group	10%
	vegetable group	15%
	fluids	10%

Figure 31-2A–B Alternate methods of documenting meal intake.

FLUID BALANCE

Fluid balance is the balance between liquid intake and liquid output. The metric system is used for fluid measurements: milliliters (ml) or cubic centimeters (cc). A milliliter and a cubic centimeter are the same amount.

Intake

We take in approximately 2.5 quarts (2,500 ml) of fluid daily. Most adult patients will need to consume an average 600 to 800 ml of fluid during each 8-hour shift. Excessive fluid retention is called edema. Inadequate fluid intake results in dehydration, or the lack of sufficient fluid in body tissues. Some disease conditions may change the amount of fluids the patient is allowed to have.

Typical output equals about 2.5 quarts daily in the form of:

- Urine, 1.5 quarts (1,500 mL)
- Perspiration
- Moisture from the lungs
- Moisture from the bowel

Excessive fluid loss results in dehydration. This can occur through:

- Diarrhea
- Vomiting
- Excessive urine output (diuresis)
- Excessive perspiration (diaphoresis)
- Inadequate fluid intake

Recording Intake and Output

An accurate recording of intake and output (I&O), or fluid taken in and given off by the body, is basic to the care of many patients. Intake and output records are kept when specifically ordered by the physician or registered nurse.

Pushing Fluids

Fluid intake may need to be encouraged in some patients. This is called push fluids or force fluids. In some situations (as in kidney disease), fluid intake may have to be restricted. Fluid intake and output are calculated by measuring and recording the fluids the patient takes in and the fluids the patient excretes (eliminates from the body). Because the fluids taken in by the patient cannot actually be measured, an estimate is made and recorded.

This is done by:

• Knowing what the liquid container holds when full

• Estimating how much is gone from the container (what the patient drank), such as one-third of a glass of juice or half a cup of coffee

• Converting this to milliliters (e.g., a water glass holds 240 mL when filled; the patient drinks three-fourths of the glass of water; $\frac{3}{4} \times 240 = 180$ mL)

Fluid Consumption

• You should know whether a patient is allowed ice or tap water and if water is to be especially encouraged.

• Encourage all patients to take six to eight glasses of fluids daily, unless the patient is NPO (nothing by mouth) or on restricted fluids.

• Give special attention to confused patients, patients who may not be able to reach a source of water, and the elderly.

• When "force fluids" is ordered, encourage the patient to drink each time you are in the room.

• Offer to assist, if necessary. Some patients will not drink water.

• Find out what beverages the patient likes and provide these, if possible.

FEEDING THE PATIENT

Eating should be an enjoyable experience. Prepare the patient for his or her tray before it arrives.

When you have served the tray and after you have washed your hands, assist the patient as needed. If the patient cannot see, explain the arrangement of the tray as if the items on it were on the face of a clock.

Note: Carry some extra straws with you during meal times. It can save you steps.

Assisting Patients Who Have Swallowing Problems

Patients who have difficulty swallowing may require one-to-one assistance, prompting, or supervision at meals. The speech therapist recommends special techniques and positions for improving swallowing and preventing choking. These will be listed on the care plan.

• Before serving food or beverages, make sure the patient is fully awake and alert.

• Position the patient in the upright position.

• The head should face forward, with the body flexed forward slightly.

• Avoid tipping the head back, which increases the risk of choking.

• During the meal, reduce distractions.

• Focus the patient on eating.

• Prompt or feed the patient slowly, offering small bites.

• Remind him or her to chew the food well.

• Check the care plan for additional directions.

ALTERNATIVE NUTRITION

Total Parenteral Nutrition

Total parenteral nutrition (TPN) is a technique in which high-density

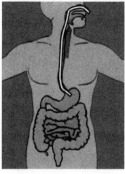 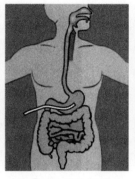 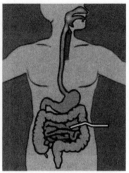

A. Nasogastric route   B. Gastrostomy route   C. Jejunostomy route

Figure 31-3 Enteral feeding methods: (A) Nasogastric feeding; (B) Gastrostomy feeding; (C) Jejunostomy feeding.

(concentrated) nutrients are introduced into a large vein such as the subclavian vein or the superior vena cava. This method of feeding is used for patients who have diseases of the digestive tract.

Enteral Feedings

Enteral feedings may be administered by a tube that is:

- Inserted through the nose and into the stomach (*nasogastric*, or NG, feeding)
- Placed surgically, such as the *gastrostomy* (*G-tube or GT*) (Figure 31-3B) and *percutaneous endoscopic gastrostomy* (*PEG*) tube.
  - The PEG is surgically inserted by threading the tube through the mouth and into the stomach, then it is pulled out through an incision in the abdomen. Tubes that have been surgically placed are initially covered with a dressing. After the insertion site has healed, the area is usually left uncovered.
- For special purposes, such as the *jejunostomy tube* (*J-tube*) (Figure 31-3C). J-tubes are used for patients who do not have a stomach,

and those in whom recurrent formula aspiration is a problem. This is a very long, small-bore tube that is threaded through the GI tract until the tip reaches the small intestine. Occasionally, you may see a J-tube that has been placed through the nose (nasojejunostomy), but these are less common. The most common J-tube is surgically inserted through an incision in the abdominal skin. This is considered to be a long-term tube.

When caring for the patient with tube feedings, you must:

- Keep the head of the bed elevated 30 to 45 degrees during feeding and for 30 to 60 minutes after feeding.
- Check the taping of tubes. If tape is loose, pulls, or is causing skin irritation, inform the nurse.
- Report any retching, nausea, or vomiting immediately.
- Check tubing for kinks. Be sure patient is not lying on tubing.
- Provide frequent mouth hygiene.
- Notify nurse if controlling device alarm sounds.
- Avoid pulling the tubing when moving the patient.

CHAPTER

WARM AND COLD APPLICATIONS

32

Heat and cold applications are used only on written orders from the physician or nurse for a specified length of time. *Some states have laws against nursing assistants applying heat or cold in a home health setting.* In other facilities, nursing assistants who have been specially trained are permitted to carry out these procedures under the supervision of the nurse. Be sure you know and follow the policy of your facility and are adequately prepared and supervised.

THERAPY WITH HEAT AND COLD

The physician orders the use of heat and cold applications. Applications of warm and cold may be either dry or moist. Moisture makes both heat and cold more penetrating. Therefore, moist heat or moist cold is more likely to cause injury. Extra care must be taken to protect the patient when moist treatments are used. Be sure you know:

- Exact method to be used
- Correct temperature and placement
- Proper length of time the warm or cold application is to be performed
- How often the area being treated is to be checked

Guidelines for Warm and Cold Treatments

You must be very watchful when applying cold or warm treatments. When assigned to this task, keep in mind the following:

- The age and condition of the patient. Give extra care to:
  - Young children
  - The aged
  - Patients with cognitive impairment
  - Patients who are uncooperative
  - Patients who are unconscious
  - Patients who are paralyzed
  - Patients with tissue damage
  - Patients with poor circulation
- An electric heating pad must not be used with moist dressings unless a rubber cover is placed over the pad. If the wires become damp, a short circuit may result. The patient must not lie on the pad, because severe burns can result. Sensitivity to heat varies, so patients receiving heat treatments must be checked frequently. Although heating pads are not used in health care facilities, they are used by individuals in homes.
- Heat is not applied to the head because it could make blood vessels in the area dilate, causing headaches.
- Heat should not be applied to the abdomen if there is any chance that the patient has appendicitis, because it would increase the chance of the appendix rupturing.
- Areas where cold treatments are used should be carefully and frequently checked for discoloration and numbness. If the area is discolored or numb, discontinue the treatment and report to the nurse.

- Rubber or plastic should never touch the patient's skin. Be sure all appliances are covered with cloth.

Use of Cold Applications

Applications of cold are given only with a physician's order. See Table 32-1.

Cautions

- Excessive cold can damage body tissues.
- Report color changes such as *blanching* (turning white) or *cyanosis* (becoming bluish).
- Report feelings of numbness or discomfort experienced by patient.
- Stop the cold treatment if the patient starts to shiver. Cover the patient with a blanket and report immediately to the nurse.

Cold therapy should not be used for patients with:
- Deep vein thrombosis
- Peripheral vascular disease
- Open wound(s)
- Skin sensation impairment

- Severe cognitive impairment
- Cold intolerance, cold allergy
- Some medical conditions such as rheumatoid arthritis and Reynaud's phenomenon

If a patient has any of these conditions, check with the nurse before using a cold application.

Dry Cold Applications

Careful attention to application is needed to prevent injury. When using disposable cold packs, follow the manufacturer's directions exactly. When activating the pack, do not hold it in front of your face. If the pack leaks or bursts, the chemicals inside it may splash. Check the area being treated every 10 minutes. Do not attempt to refreeze the cold pack.

Moist Cold Applications

Wet compresses are moistened with a solution and placed on the affected area.
- A syringe may be used to add water to the compresses to keep them moist.

Table 32-1   AVERAGE ORDERED TEMPERATURES FOR HEAT AND COLD TREATMENTS AND PROCEDURES

HOT 100°F to 105°F

Warm 95°F to 100°F (This is the range that is used for bathing and most treatments; the highest comfortable bath temperature is about 105°F.)

For some procedures, you may be instructed to prepare water at a temperature of 110°F. This is because the water is expected to cool before the patient uses the treatment. Temperatures should never exceed 105°F when they are applied to the patient or when the patient's body is immersed in water.

Tepid 80°F to 95°F

Cool 65°F to 80°F

Cold 45°F to 65°F

- Never set the whirlpool for higher than 100°F without first checking with the RN. (The whirlpool is preset to maintain a constant temperature of 97°F. Because it maintains a constant temperature, it should not need adjustment.)

- These guidelines may also be appropriate for other treatments; facility policies and the RN's directions supercede the information given here.

- The compresses may be kept cold by placing a covered ice bag against the affected area.
- Each time the pad is removed and replaced, be careful to reposition the protective covering.

Follow facility policy for:
- Method of applying the treatment
- Length of time treatment is to be applied
- How often patient is to be checked for condition of skin in the treatment area and general response to the treatment
- Signs that treatment should be discontinued

Use of Warm Applications

The value of heat treatments is that heat dilates or increases the size of blood vessels, which brings more blood to the area to promote healing. Warmth is very soothing when there is pain. There must be a specific order for a warm application. See Table 32-1.

Cautions

Follow these cautions when working with patients:
- Constant warmth must be carefully monitored.
- Moisture intensifies the effect of warmth. Use extra caution.
- Hot packs are contraindicated in paralysis or areas without sensation, acute edema or inflammation, infection, and hemophilia. They must be used with caution in many medical conditions, including in patients with impaired circulation, sensory impairment, cancer, and rashes and open skin conditions, and in very young or very old patients.
- Never allow a patient to lie on a constant heat unit, because heat may be trapped and build up to dangerous levels.

- The temperature of a constant heat unit should be between 95° and 100°F.
- Always use a bath thermometer to check solution temperatures.
- Always remove the body part being soaked before adding warm solution.
- Always stay with the patient during the treatment.
- Protect areas not being treated from excessive exposure.
- Warmth is not applied to the head because it could cause blood vessels in the area to dilate, resulting in headaches.
- Rubber or plastic should never touch the patient's skin. Be sure all appliances are covered in cloth.

Heat therapy should not be used for patients with:
- Acute inflammation
- Dermatitis
- Deep vein thrombosis
- Peripheral vascular disease
- Open wound(s)
- Recent soft tissue injuries in which swelling or bleeding would be increased by heat
- Skin sensation impairment
- Severe cognitive impairment

Some physicians also recommend avoiding heat in children and women during pregnancy. If a patient has any of these conditions, check with the nurse before applying a heat application.

For each of the warm treatments, follow the facility policy for:
- Method of applying the treatment
- Length of time treatment is to be applied
- How often the patient is to be checked for condition of skin in the treatment area and general response to treatment

- Signs that treatment should be discontinued

TEMPERATURE CONTROL MEASURES

Excessively high or low temperatures are treated in acute care facilities by placing hypothermia-hyperthermia blankets under the patient. These blankets are filled with water, and the temperature of the water can be adjusted.

Immediately notify the nurse if you observe any of these complications:
- Changes in skin color
- Cyanosis of the lips or nail beds
- Sudden changes in temperature
- Marked changes in pulse, respirations, and blood pressure
- Respiratory distress
- Pain
- Changes in sensation
- Edema
- Shivering and chills
- Urinary output below 50 ml/hour

After removing the blanket, continue checking vital signs and intake and output every 30 minutes for the first 2 hours, then hourly or as directed by the nurse.

Hypothermia

Hypothermia is a drop in core body temperature below 95°F (35°C) rectally. Indications of hypothermia to report include:
- Drop in body temperature
- Poor coordination and confusion
- Slurred speech
- Decreased respiratory and heart rates

Nursing Assistant Actions
- Report observations to the nurse.

- Check the environmental temperature and adjust it.
- Provide external warmth with a sweater or blanket.
- Reduce drafts with screens or curtains.
- If permitted, give something warm to drink.
- Check vital signs.

Hyperthermia

Hyperthermia is an elevation of core body temperature to 104°F (40°C) or higher rectally. Indications of hyperthermia to report include:
- Elevated body temperature
- Hot, flushed skin
- Faintness
- Headache
- Nausea
- Convulsions

Fever, or *pyrexia,* is when the core body temperature rises to at least 101°F rectally. In children, temperatures tend to rise higher than in adults. This puts children at greater risk for seizures.

Nursing Assistant Actions
- Report observations to the nurse.
- Check environmental temperature and adjust it.
- Reduce external warmth. Cover the patient only with a gown or sheet.
- If permitted, give a cooling drink.
- Carry out cooling procedures as ordered. For example, give cooling baths or enemas.
- Check vital signs frequently.

THE SURGICAL PATIENT

33

PREOPERATIVE CARE

You may answer general questions that the patient asks, but you must refer specific questions about the surgery, its possible outcome, and anesthesia to the nurse. It is helpful if you are aware of the information that has been given to the patient.

Psychological Preparation

Because you will be in frequent contact with the patient, you may be the first person to recognize signs of fear or concern. Listen to what the patient says and observe his or her body language carefully. Report your observations to the nurse so that appropriate nursing intervention can be carried out.

Physical Preparation

The Surgical Prep Area

Skin preparation before surgery may or may not include hair removal. There is a trend away from removing hair unless its thickness will interfere with the surgery. Some studies have shown more infections among shaved patients than among unshaved patients.

If shaving is ordered, it must be done according to the procedure provided. It must be performed skillfully in a well-lighted area. The area to be washed and shaved will be larger than the surgical incision area. See Figure 33-1.

To prepare the surgical area by shaving:
- Make sure you know exactly what area is to be shaved. Most hospitals have routine prep areas.
- Do not shave the neck or face of a female patient. If in doubt, check with the nurse.
- Never shave the eyebrows.
- Be aware that the preparations for cranial surgery are usually performed after the patient has been medicated and taken to the operating suite. Doctors have special preferences in this regard.
- Remember that if a spinal anesthetic is to be given, the back may also be shaved.

Caution: All personnel involved in the perioperative care of the patient must be alert to make sure that the correct surgical procedure is done on the correct patient, and that the surgery is done on the correct site. This often involves marking the site of surgery. Various forms and checklists are used to verify the patient and surgical site. Take your responsibilities for identifying the patient and operative site seriously. There is no room for error.

Immediate Preoperative Care

Approximately 1 hour before surgery, the patient will be given additional medication by the nurse. Your responsibilities regarding the patient must be completed before

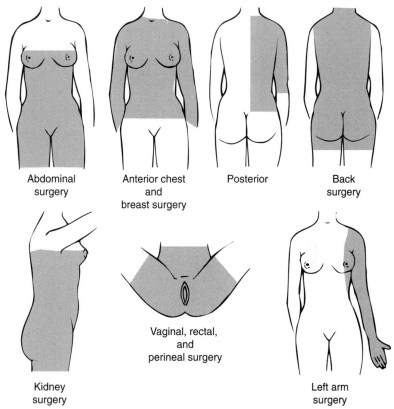

Abdominal surgery

Anterior chest and breast surgery

Posterior

Back surgery

Vaginal, rectal, and perineal surgery

Kidney surgery

Left arm surgery

Figure 33-1 Hair is removed preoperatively within each of the shaded areas upon physicians' order.

this time. You may be asked to do the following:

- Take and record vital signs.
- Take care of valuables according to hospital policy. Remove dentures and any other prosthesis (artificial part) such as a hearing aid or glasses. See that they are safely marked with the patient's name and cared for.
- Remove nail polish, makeup, hairpins, and jewelry. Long hair should be neatly braided or capped. Plain wedding bands may be taped in place.

- Dress the patient in a gown and cover the hair with a surgical cap.
- See that the patient voids and measure the urine. Drain catheter bag, if present.
- Make sure that the room is quiet and comfortable.

As soon as the nurse gives the preoperative medication:

- Be sure the side rails are in place for safety.
  - Do not let the patient get up to use the bathroom unassisted. Provide the bedpan or urinal, if necessary.

- Remove all unnecessary equipment.
- Push the bedside table, overbed table, and chair out of the way to make room for the stretcher when it arrives from surgery.
- Complete the surgical checklist.
- Follow facility policy regarding visitors. Sometimes they are allowed to wait quietly with the patient. Sometimes they need to be directed to the visitors' waiting room.
- Elevate the bed to stretcher height when the transporter arrives to take the patient to surgery.

You will probably be asked to assist in transferring the patient from the bed to the stretcher and, after surgery, from the stretcher to the bed.

DURING THE OPERATIVE PERIOD

While the patient is in the operating room, you will prepare the room for his or her return.
- A surgical bed will be prepared. This is also called a postop or recovery bed.
- Everything should be moved from the top of the bedside stand except an emesis basin, tissue wipes, tongue depressors, and equipment to check vital signs.
- Necessary documentation on which to record vital signs should also be available.
- Check with the nurse for any special equipment, such as oxygen, IV poles, suction, or drainage bags, that might be necessary for your patient.
- While carrying out your other assignments, be watchful for the return of your patient from surgery.
- Follow facility policy regarding the location of visitors and family during surgery.

POSTOPERATIVE CARE

When the patient's condition is stabilized, the patient is returned to the unit. Upon the patient's return from the recovery room, you should:
- Identify the patient.
- Assist in the transfer from stretcher to bed.
- Never leave the unconscious patient alone at any time.
- Check with the nurse for special instructions to be followed.
- Realize that the patient may be drowsy for several hours after return.
- Have an extra blanket available— many patients complain of feeling cold upon return.

Remember that most patients receive many drugs with the potential to alter their mental status when they are in surgery. The drugs are excreted slowly from the body. The patient may sleep soundly upon return to the unit. Keep the side rails up and follow all safety precautions until the patient is fully awake and the nurse instructs you that side rails are no longer necessary. Do not leave liquids at the bedside until the nurse instructs you that it is safe to do so. Check on the patient regularly.

During the perioperative period, many factors interfere with the patient's normal temperature-regulating mechanisms. Normally, we shiver when we are cold. The blood vessels constrict. *Perioperative hypothermia* develops in the operating room. Anesthesia and some sedatives disrupt the internal ability to regulate temperature. The drugs promote heat loss by reducing the shivering response and preventing blood vessel constriction. Underlying factors such as age, presence of chronic disease, and body size also affect temperature regulation. Open body cavities and administration of blood and IV fluids further contribute to temperature loss.

The body cannot return the temperature to normal until the concentration of anesthetic in the brain decreases and the normal temperature regulating responses are triggered and can take over. Pain further decreases the effectiveness of these responses. Because of these factors, return to normal temperature may take two to five hours, depending on the degree of hypothermia and the age of the patient. Perioperative outcomes are better if the patient does not become hypothermic. Notify the nurse promptly if the patient has a low body temperature or the temperature does not progressively increase with your routine vital sign checks. Monitor for shivering, complaints of feeling cold, and cold skin temperature and inform the nurse.

Nursing Assistant Responsibilities

The following are routine instructions to be followed unless otherwise ordered:

- Always wear gloves and follow standard precautions when contact with blood, body fluids, mucous membranes, or nonintact skin is likely.
- Take vital signs of the patient upon arrival on the unit and every 15 minutes for four readings. The patient's temperature may not always be taken at this time. When taking postoperative vital signs, count pulse and respirations for 1 full minute. Most facilities have policies for postoperative vital signs at specified frequencies that decrease if the vital signs are stable (approximately the same), such as:

  - Every 15 minutes for 1 hour
  - If stable, every 30 minutes for 1 hour
  - If stable, every hour for 2 hours
  - If stable, every 4 hours for 24 hours
- Monitor the patient's level of consciousness (drowsy, unresponsive, alert) each time you check the vital signs.
- Anesthesia reduces body temperature.
- Keep the patient warm.
- If the patient's temperature is below 97°F, inform the nurse promptly.
- Check dressings for amount and type of any drainage.
- Check IV solutions for flow rate. Restrain infusion site whenever ordered.
- Encourage the patient to breathe deeply, cough, and move in bed. Position should be changed every 2 hours.
- If the patient is vomiting, turn his or her head to one side and support it. Have an emesis basin ready, as well as tissues and wet cloth. If the patient is conscious, allow him or her to rinse mouth with water after vomiting. Note type and amount of vomitus and record on the output worksheet.
- Check pulses distal to the operative site. Inform the nurse if the pulse is weak or cannot be felt.
- If the patient was given a spinal anesthetic:
  - Give extra care in turning frequently and maintaining proper alignment.
  - Remember the patient will be unable to move independently until sensation and motor functions return. Make sure to calm the patient's fear about this.
  - Some physicians require that the patient remain flat on the back

and without a pillow for 8 to 12 hours following spinal anesthesia to avoid headaches.

- Any complaints of a headache following spinal anesthesia should be reported promptly.
- Provide extra blankets if the patient is cold.

• Be sure all drainage tubes have been connected (the nurse will usually attend to this). If you notice a tube clamped shut, check with the nurse.

• Measure and record the first postoperative voiding. Inform the nurse.

• Report any patient complaints of discomfort and pain to the nurse.

• Since many facilities consider pain to be the fifth vital sign, you should ask the patient if he or she is having pain each time you check the vital signs. If pain is present, inform the nurse.

Tubes

The following are some special precautions to be taken:

• Always wear gloves if contact with drainage from the tube is likely.

• Learn the type, purpose, and location of each tube.

• Check drainage for character and amount.

• Check for obstructions to the tube system.

• Check flow rate of infusions from intravenous lines.

• Keep orifices (body openings) clear of secretions and discharge.

• Never disconnect tubes or raise drainage bottles above the level of the drainage site.

• Never lower infusion bottles below the level of the infusion site.

• Never put stress on the tubes when moving the patient or giving care.

• Restrain infusion sites as necessary to prevent dislocation.

Note: A physician's order is needed.

• Monitor levels of infusions and report to the nurse before they run out.

• Report any signs of leakage or disconnected tubes immediately.

• Report pain, discoloration, or swelling at sites of drainage or infusion.

Drainage

When a body cavity is the operative site, it may be necessary to drain fluid such as blood, pus, serous drainage caused by tissue trauma, or gastric contents from it before or after surgery. Always wear gloves if contact with drainage is likely.

Body sites with tubes, drains, and surgical dressings are managed using sterile technique. Never open a tube or drain or remove a dressing. Some drains cause drainage to accumulate on the dressing. You should:

• Note the amount and character of the drainage.

• Inform the nurse when the dressing needs to be changed or reinforced.

At times, the withdrawal of fluids is controlled by attaching the drainage tube to a connecting tube and then a suction apparatus. The drainage accumulates in a container. The container is emptied and the contents measured at the end of the shift.

It is your responsibility to:

• Report either light or heavy drainage.

• Report a change in the character or amount of the drainage.

• Make sure that the flow of drainage is not blocked by kinking of the tube.

Never assume responsibility for chest drainage or attempt to empty chest bottles. Chest bottles and irrigations require the nurse's or physician's attention.

The patient must be carefully observed, especially during the first 24 hours, for possible complications. Possible postoperative discomfort and complications and appropriate nursing assistant actions are summarized in Table 33-1.

When the patient has responded sufficiently and vital signs are stable, he or she may be refreshed by:
• Washing the hands and face
• Changing the linen
• Being given a light backrub

Deep Breathing and Coughing

Deep breathing and coughing clear the air passages. This may be an uncomfortable task when the patient has a new incision. Assist the patient by:
• Explaining the value of the exercise.
• Assisting the patient to deep breathe and cough.
• Checking with the nurse to see if medication for pain is to be administered before the exercise. If so, wait for 45 minutes after the medication has been given before carrying out the exercise.
• Learning from the nurse how many deep breaths and coughs should be attempted. The usual number is 5 to 10 breaths and 2 to 3 coughs.
• Using a pillow or binder to support the incision during the procedure.

Although we routinely encourage postoperative patients to cough and deep breathe, there are a few exceptions you must be aware of. Avoid this procedure with patients who have had eye, nose, or neurologic surgery. Coughing and deep breathing will increase pressure, causing complications in these patients. Check with the nurse if you are unsure of what action to take.

Apply the principles of standard precautions when assisting with coughing and deep breathing procedures. If the patient is expelling loose secretions, select and wear appropriate protective equipment, including gloves, gown, mask, and face shield. Show the patient how to contain secretions in tissue. Assist him or her with handwashing after the activity.

Leg Exercises

Leg exercises following surgery encourage steady circulation. This helps to prevent another serious complication of the postoperative period—the development of blood clots.

A specific order must be written for leg exercises when there has been surgery on the legs themselves. Otherwise, leg exercises are performed routinely by the patient. If the patient is very weak, you may need to assist.
• Encourage leg exercises and be sure they have been performed.
• Each exercise should be performed at least three to five times every 1 or 2 hours and at other times as well.
• Carry out leg exercises as you assist position changes.
• Apply or reapply support hose (TED) after exercises if ordered.

Elasticized Stockings

Elasticized stockings, called TED hose or antiembolism hose, that extend from the ankle or foot to calf or midthigh are often ordered. This reduces the incidence of thrombophlebitis, which is inflammation of the veins that can lead to blood clots. The stockings must be applied smoothly and evenly before the patient gets out of bed. They should be removed and reapplied at least every 8 hours—more often if necessary or as ordered.

Several types of antiembolism hose are used. Some have closed toes, but

Table 33-1 POSTOPERATIVE COMPLICATIONS AND NURSING ASSISTANT ACTIONS

POSSIBLE DISCOMFORT	REPORT	WHAT YOU CAN DO*
Thirst	Patient complaints of dryness of lips, mouth, and skin	Carefully check I&O. Give ice chips or increase fluid intake by mouth with permission. Monitor IV if ordered. Give mouth care. Check blood pressure and pulse. Watch for signs of shock and hemorrhage.
Singultus (hiccups)—intermittent spasms of the diaphragm	Incidence of hiccups	Allow patient to rest; hiccups can be tiring. Support incisional area. Assist patient to breathe into paper bag.
Pain	Location, intensity, type	Change position. Apply warmth if instructed. Monitor carefully for and report effects of medication given by nurse.
Distention (accumulation of gas in bowel)	Distention of abdomen, complaints of pain	Increase mobility. Insert a rectal tube if instructed and permitted.
Nausea, vomiting	Nausea, character of vomitus	Keep emesis basin at bedside. Monitor IV fluids, which are substituted for oral fluids. Give mouth care. Limit fluids by mouth. Record the amount of vomitus as output on the I&O record. Encourage patient to breathe deeply.
Urinary retention	Amount and time of first voiding. Distention, restlessness, imbalance between I&O	Monitor I&O carefully. Check for distention.

Complication	Signs and Symptoms	Action
Hemorrhage (excessive blood loss)	Fall in blood pressure; cold, moist skin; weak, rapid pulse; restlessness; pallor/cyanosis; condition of dressing; thirst	Report immediately to nurse. Keep patient quiet. Check vital signs.
Shock	Fall in blood pressure; weak, rapid pulse; cold, moist skin; pallor	Report immediately to nurse. Keep patient quiet. Monitor ordered oxygen. Be prepared to follow additional instructions.
Hypoxia (lack of oxygen)	Restlessness, dyspnea, crowing sounds to respirations, pounding pulse, perspiration	Report immediately to nurse. Monitor oxygen, if ordered.
Atelectasis (failure of lungs to expand)	Dyspnea; cyanosis/pallor	Report immediately to nurse.
Wound infection	Increased pain in incisional area; fever; chills, anorexia, increased drainage on dressing	Be observant. Report findings promptly to nurse. Check dressing.
Wound disruption (separation of wound edges)	Pinkish drainage; complaints by the patient that he or she "feels open," "broken," "giving way"	Report immediately to nurse. Keep patient quiet. Support incisional area.
Pulmonary emboli	Anxiety, difficulty breathing; feelings of "heaviness in chest," cyanosis, chest pain	Keep patient quiet. Report immediately to nurse. Elevate head of bed.

*In all cases, be prepared to follow the nurse's additional instructions.

most have an opening near the toe end. The hole is positioned on the top or bottom of the foot, just proximal to the toes. Check the heel placement on the stocking. By using the heel as a landmark, you will see where to position the hole in the stocking.

Sequential Compression Therapy

Deep vein thrombosis and pulmonary embolus (blood clot in the lungs) are serious postoperative complications. Approximately 10% of all patients with DVT die from pulmonary embolus. Most have no symptoms until they develop the embolus. The femoral vein, the large blood vessel in the groin, is particularly susceptible to clot formation. Because of the high risk and serious consequences associated with blood clots, the physician may order sequential compression therapy to reduce the risk.

Pneumatic hosiery, also called sequential compression hosiery, prevents blood clots by massaging the legs with a milking, wavelike motion. Pneumatic hosiery inflates and deflates rhythmically. The device should not be used on patients with lower leg ulcers, blood clots, massive edema, deformities, infected or broken skin, or arterial disease. Shiny, hairless skin is an indication of arterial problems. If you observe any hard nodules or red or warm areas on the patient's lower legs, inform the nurse before applying any hosiery.

Before applying the hosiery, palpate the pedal and posterior tibial pulses. Compare the movement, sensation, and color in both feet. If abnormalities are noted, consult the nurse before continuing. The nurse will evaluate the patient's legs and check for contraindications. Follow his or her instructions.

Follow your facility policy for documenting the use of the pneumatic compression device. You may be asked to document the procedure, pulse checks in the feet, skin color, the patient's response, and the settings, including use of the alarm and cooling settings.

Initial Ambulation

Sometime after surgery, a patient is permitted to sit up with the legs over the edge of the bed. This position is called dangling.

- Watch carefully for signs of fatigue or dizziness (vertigo).
- Assist the patient to assume the position slowly.

The first ambulation (walk) is usually short. The patient usually dangles for a short time before ambulating. Dangling is also an important part of postoperative care because it stimulates circulation and helps prevent the formation of blood clots (thrombi).

Remain next to the patient during the first dangling and ambulation. For patient safety, do not turn your back or leave the bedside. Use common sense, and follow the care plan and the nurse's instructions.

The patient may need assistance the first few times he or she stands up to ambulate. The anesthetic and medications administered before, during, and after surgery may affect the patient's balance, endurance, and strength. There may be drainage tubes or an intravenous feeding that must be moved with the patient.

Guidelines for Assisting the Patient in Initial Ambulation

- Check with the nurse to see if a transfer belt can be used.

- Assist the patient to sit on the edge of the bed with bed in low position.
- Assist the patient to put on footwear appropriate to the floor surface. Never allow a patient to ambulate with bare feet or socks.
- Take the patient's pulse before and after standing. If there is more than a 10-point difference, return the patient to bed and inform the nurse.
- If the patient becomes dizzy or faint, return him or her to bed and inform the nurse.
- Walk with the patient following facility policy.

CARING FOR THE EMOTIONALLY STRESSED PATIENT

34

PROFESSIONAL BOUNDARIES

As a nursing assistant, you must stay within certain *professional boundaries* when caring for each patient. Boundaries are unspoken limits on physical and emotional relationship with patients. They limit and define how a worker acts with patients. Boundaries are invisible, and you must use good judgment and common sense to identify them and avoid crossing them. Boundary violations are a potential problem with all patients, but have enhanced potential for repercussions when working with mental health patients.

Boundary violations lead to inappropriate relationships with patients or families that may cloud your clinical judgment. Violations often lead to serious consequences, and usually carry over into your personal life. You may do things you would not normally do. For your own well-being, be aware that professional boundaries exist and actively take steps to keep from crossing them.

To avoid crossing professional boundaries, strive to act professionally, as you were taught in class. Avoid putting yourself in a position in which you think and act as a family member or friend. You must use good judgment and determine the amount of contact and assistance that are right for the patient. Too much or too little contact can be unhealthy

for you and the patient. Review the complete information on boundaries in Unit 30 of your text. Consult the nurse or another professional you can trust if you are uncertain.

Ethical Behavior with Patients and Families

As a nursing assistant, patients expect you to act in their best interests and treat them with dignity. You do this by not taking advantage of a patient's situation and avoiding inappropriate involvement with the patient and his or her family. It is not always easy to recognize unhealthy relationships until it is too late. Once you have crossed a boundary line, turning back may be difficult. Be aware of boundaries at all times, and strive to keep your relationships professional. Avoid:

- thinking you are immune from having unhealthy relationships.
- discussing your personal problems with patients or their families.
- being flirtatious with a patient, or displaying behavior that could be misinterpreted.
- discussing feelings of sexual attraction with a patient.
- putting yourself in a position in which you are at risk of having a sexual relationship with a patient.
- keeping secrets with a patient.
- becoming defensive when someone questions your involvement with a patient.

216

- believing that you are the only nursing assistant who can meet the patient's needs.
- spending an inappropriate amount of time with a patient.
- visiting a patient when you are off duty.
- trading assignments with others to be with a patient.
- failing to report or reporting only partial information about a patient to the nurse because you fear disclosing negative information or secrets the patient has told you.
- feeling that you must protect the patient from other workers.
- always siding with the patient's position.

Enabling

Enabling behavior is shielding a person from experiencing the full impact or consequences of his or her behavior. It differs from helping behavior because it allows the person to be irresponsible. It is easy to be manipulated into an enabling situation by a patient. Learning, respecting, and adhering to professional boundaries will help you avoid helping others inappropriately. You should also learn to set limits for yourself and keep patients from crossing into your own personal space or boundaries. Enabling behavior creates dependency. It does not help move the patient toward independence and good mental health. Methods of enabling patients that you should avoid include:

- protecting the patient from the natural consequences of his or her behavior;
- keeping secrets about a patient's behavior from others;
- making excuses for a patient's behavior;
- acting to get a patient out of personal trouble;
- blaming others for the patient's behavior;
- seeing the patient's problems as a result of something or someone else;
- giving money to patients;
- attempting to control patients lives and activities; and
- doing things for the patient that she should do herself.

Strive to keep your behavior in the zone of helpfulness (Figure 34-1) to avoid crossing professional boundaries and enabling patients.

MENTAL HEALTH DISORDERS

A variety of like conditions are grouped together into several mental health categories. A summary of common categories is listed here.

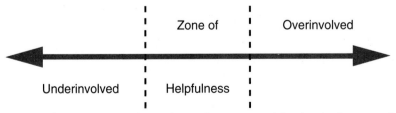

Figure 34-1 Keep your relationship with patients and families in the zone of helpfulness.

Anxiety Disorders

Anxiety disorders are conditions in which patients have signs and symptoms of anxiety in response to stress. These include:

- *Generalized anxiety* (the most common condition)—the patient has fear, apprehension, or feels a sense of impending doom. Physical symptoms, such as tension, restlessness, and rapid heart rate, may also be present.

- *Panic disorder*—characterized by unexpected, chronic *panic attacks,* or bouts of overwhelming fear. The person feels he or she is in danger without reason. The fear may be so debilitating that the person cannot function normally. Panic attacks recur, and the person worries about the next attack in between attacks.

- *Obsessive-compulsive disorder (OCD)*—an anxiety disorder in which the patient has recurrent obsessions, frequent thoughts, ideas, impulses, or compulsions, resulting in ritualistic activity over which the person has no control. He or she derives no pleasure from the ritualistic behavior. An *obsession* is an idea, impulse, or thought that usually does not make sense, but the person cannot suppress or eliminate it. He or she usually feels a sense of urgency to act on this thought. Resisting causes even more stress. A *compulsion* is a purposeful, repetitive behavior that is done many times each day and is problematic. The compulsion causes stress and interferes with the person's life. Patients with this condition may be very superstitious. For example, the person washes the hands many times each day for no reason. He or she may also hoard items, clean over and over, check and recheck something (such as seeing whether the coffee pot is turned off or the door is locked), sorting items, silently counting or repeating words or phrases, or always stepping over cracks in the sidewalk or tile floor.

- *Posttraumatic stress disorder (PTSD)*—having unusual symptoms after a stressful or traumatic event. Onset of problems may not occur until months or years after the event. The person may have nightmares or flashbacks, have trouble with normal emotional responses, feel anxious and detached from others, and have difficulty sleeping, remembering, or concentrating.

- *Phobias*—unfounded, recurring fear of an object, insect, activity, or situation that causes the person to feel panic. The phobia is almost always unreasonable. The person's reaction ranges from dread to terror, or having outright panic that may include shaking or crying. Phobias can range in severity from being mildly annoying to severely disabling.

Agitation

Agitation is defined as inappropriate verbal, vocal, or motor activity due to causes other than disorientation or real need. It includes behavior such as:

- Aimless wandering
- Pacing
- Cursing
- Screaming
- Repeatedly asking the same questions
- Spitting
- Biting
- Fighting or arguing constantly
- Demanding attention
- Restlessness

Agitation is a significant problem for the elderly, their families, and the nursing staff. It is probably one of the foremost management problems in acute care hospitals, home care, and long-term care facilities.

The major factors contributing to agitation are:

- Noise
- Frustration at loss of control
- Feelings that the patient's space has been invaded
- Loneliness and need for attention
- Unresolved personal difficulties in the patient's past
- Drug interactions
- Organic brain disease
- Boredom
- Behavior of others around the patient
- Depression
- Constipation
- Restraints
- Too much sensory stimulation

Paranoia

Paranoia is another extreme maladaptive response to stress. It is characterized by a heightened, false sense of self-importance and delusions of being persecuted. Delusions are false beliefs about oneself, other people, and events. People with paranoia believe that everyone is against them. When treating the paranoid patient, you should:

- Find ways to reduce the patient's feelings of insecurity and misunderstanding.
- Keep the person as involved as possible in reality activities.
- Report and document observed responses to medication and psychotherapy.
- Monitor nutrition and fluid balance—these patients often refuse to eat or drink for fear of poisoning.

- Observe sleep patterns—the person may be fearful of being harmed while sleeping.
- Be direct and honest in all interactions.
- Not support any misconceptions or delusions that the person exhibits.
- Never argue with anyone who has delusions. It can trigger a serious confrontation.

ASSISTING PATIENTS TO COPE

Here are some ways to help patients become better able to cope and adapt:

- Be a good listener.
- Try to determine the source of stress so it can be removed and the stress reduced.
- Be sensitive to body language that may give clues to the source of stress.
- Treat the person with respect, recognizing him or her as a unique individual.
- Try to understand the behavior in the same way the patient is viewing it, without labeling the behavior and passing judgment.
- Let the patient know you respect his or her privacy and feelings.
- Never argue, enter into a power struggle, or debate with a patient, even when you know the patient is wrong.
- Be supportive of the person's own attempts to overcome the stress.
- Remember that illness, age, and separation from family and home are major stress factors.

THE DEMANDING PATIENT

Being demanding is another way that patients express their frustration. It is a coping behavior. Patients who are very demanding are usually very frustrated by their loss of control. To be successful in caring for these patients, the nursing assistant must:

- Try to learn and understand the factors that are causing the demanding behavior.
- Show that you care about the patient's situation, but keep control of your emotions.
- Maintain open communications by listening to the patient's words and by being sensitive to the patient's body language.
- Provide opportunities that allow the patient to regain some control by making choices.
- Be consistent in your manner of care.
- Do not take the patient's demands personally.
- Report observations to the nurse with suggestions for changes in the care plan.

Patients with coping and behavior problems usually have a behavior management care plan that lists steps to follow when certain problems are exhibited. Become familiar with the care plan and implement the approaches in the order listed. Modify your behavior in response to the patient's behavior by monitoring how the patient responds to you, then adjusting your approach to achieve results. Vary routines and equipment, if necessary. Put yourself in the patient's shoes and try to understand what is happening. Inform the nurse if you identify a trigger that causes the behaviors.

Affective Disorders

Affective disorders are characterized by a disturbance in mood. They may also be called *mood disorders*, and are usually marked by a profound and persistent sadness. Depression is the most common of these disorders. Other common affective disorders are:

- *Bipolar Affective Disorder*—a disorder in which the moods swing beyond what most people experience. It may also be called *manic depression* or *bipolar depression*. Moods vary rapidly from elation (*mania*) to depression. Most people with this condition cycle between depression and mania.
- *Seasonal Affective Disorder (SAD)*— depression that recurs at the same time each year, usually starting in fall or winter and ending in spring or early summer. The cause is not known, but it is believed to be related to lack of exposure to sunlight or having abnormal melatonin levels. Some doctors treat it with light therapy.
- *Borderline Personality Disorder*—a condition in which the person is very unstable, and may be impulsive, fear abandonment, and be prone to self-injury. People with this condition can be very manipulative to family, friends, and health care workers. They have difficulty maintaining stable relationships. Although their moods are often inconsistent, they are never neutral. They usually have strong and concrete opinions, difficulty with emotional reasoning, disrupted relationships, and difficulty functioning in a way society views as normal.
- *Schizoaffective Disorder*—a combination of schizophrenia and a mood disorder that is chronic and disabling. It is difficult to diagnose. The symptoms swing from depression to delusions, hallucinations, and other signs of schizophrenia. The mood symptoms last longer than the schizophrenia.

Depression

Depression is the most common functional disorder in older people, but younger people may also experience depression. Depression may be shown in a variety of ways. Depression is often masked by symptoms that make it seem as though the patient is physically ill. Your observations are doubly important because a patient who is depressed may actually have minor or major illnesses. These infirmities may in turn cause depression. Remember, physical and mental health are interrelated.

When depression is severe, suicidal thoughts and attempts are a real possibility. You must be alert to the possibility of such a situation and report and document your observations. The suicidal patient must be carefully protected. Watch for and report:

• Change in response such as deepening depression or sudden elevation of mood
• Evidence of withdrawal or secretiveness
• Sudden loss of a support system (such as the death of a family member)
• Repeated, prolonged, or sporadic refusal of food (oral or through nasal tubes), care, medications, or fluids
• Hoarding of medication (stockpiling of pills)
• Sudden decision to donate body parts to a medical school
• Changes in behavior, especially episodes of depression, screaming, hitting, throwing things, or a sudden failure to get along with family, friends, or peers
• Sudden interest or disinterest in religion
• Purchase of a gun
• Purchase of razor blades and hiding them
• Statements such as "I just want out," "I want to end it all," "I'll never get well," "I'm going to kill myself," or "You would be better off without me"
• Increased use of alcohol and drugs
• Behavioral manifestations of anger, hostility, belligerence, loss of interest, or inability to concentrate
• Inability to do simple tasks, confusion, slurred speech, or retarded motor skills
• Deep preoccupation with something that cannot be explained

Nursing Care of a Patient with the Potential for Suicide

Never assume that a suicide attempt is a means of getting the attention of the staff or family. At least 15% of people who try to commit suicide do it again. Keep in mind that some individuals are particularly at risk. These include:

• White males over the age of 65 who live alone
• The very old (75 years and above)
• Persons with a recent diagnosis of a terminal illness
• Persons with unrelieved chronic pain
• Those suffering the sudden loss of a spouse
• The elderly with recent multiple losses

Be aware that the risk of suicide is higher on medical units than it is on surgical units. Most of the suicides occur while the patient is under the supervision of a health provider, who frequently either misses or ignores the clues of suicide. Suicide attempts may occur either when the patient is successfully recovering or is getting worse. It is the responsibility of all staff members to observe their patients carefully and immediately report any signs of depression and/or suicide. You should:

- Be observant for clues to suicide attempts and report them to the appropriate person.
- Be consistent in approaches and care.
- Encourage the patient to review his or her life, emphasizing the positive aspects.
- Give the patient hope while being realistic.
- Work to restore the person's self-esteem, self-worth, and self-respect, to preserve positive self-concept.
- Help the patient find a support network within the family, religious groups, or self-help groups.
- Make the person feel accepted as a unique, valued individual.
- Never ignore the person's threats or statements about suicide.

Guidelines for Assisting the Patient Who Is Depressed

- Reinforce the person's self-concept by emphasizing his or her continued value to society and helping the patient to use the support systems that are available.
- Do not act in a pitying way. This only validates the person's depressed feelings.
- Make sure physical supports, such as eyeglasses and hearing aids, are in place. These help the person to focus on reality.
- Report all complaints so that actual physical problems can be identified and corrected rather than being attributed to the depression.
- Provide activities, within appropriate limitations, to help the person

think beyond him- or herself. For example, engage the person in some meaningful activity such as reading, making puzzles, or conversing with others.

- Avoid tiring activities.
- Use simple language and speak slowly when giving instructions.
- Monitor elimination carefully; constipation is common.
- Provide fluids frequently, because the depressed patient may be too preoccupied to drink.
- Be alert to the potential for suicide.

Eating Disorders

Eating disorders are a group of disorders characterized by disturbances in appetite or food intake. Symptoms of these conditions overlap and are hard to identify. Eating disorders are common in patients with borderline personality disorder. Most people who suffer from eating disorders are very secretive about it, and family or close friends usually are unaware of the problem until the person appears skeletal. Medical problems and metabolic imbalances often occur, and the combination of electrolyte imbalance and starvation can lead to death. The most common eating disorders are:

- *Anorexia Nervosa*—an eating disorder in which the patient has a disturbed body image. The patient cannot maintain a minimal body weight because he believes he is fat. Most patients weigh less than 85% of the average weight for their height/sex/age. The person limits food intake, exercises vigorously, purges, and takes laxatives and diuretics. Over time, females stop having menstrual periods. Males lose interest in sex.
- *Bulimia Nervosa*—a condition in which the person consumes huge

amounts of food, then vomits (*purges*) to undo the binge. People with bulimia also use laxatives, diuretics, and vigorous exercise to lose weight. For a bulimia diagnosis, the behavior must occur at least twice a week for three months in a row. The person feels guilty, depressed, and has low self-esteem because of the binge eating.

Substance Abuse

• *Substance abuse*—a substance use disorder is characterized by the use of one or more substances (such as alcohol or drugs) that alter mood or behavior, resulting in impairment. Increased substance use often causes impaired (bad) judg-ment and maladaptive behavior that strains finances, causes irre-sponsibility, and makes the user unable to fulfill social or occupa-tional obligations. The person uses despite knowing it is dangerous or illegal to do so. Drug abuse can be by use of illegal (street) drugs or misuse of pharmaceuticals (prescription or over-the-counter drugs) without proper physician knowledge or oversight. Many individual drugs can be abused. Remember that alcohol is also considered a drug in this context. Abusers may use a single drug or combination of drugs.

Table 34-1 provides a summary of commonly abused drugs.

Table 34-1   DRUGS OF ABUSE

NAME	STREET NAME	DRUG EFFECT
Cocaine	Coke, snow, flake, crack, blow, and many others	A powerfully addictive drug that is snorted, sniffed, injected, or smoked. Crack is cocaine that has been pro-cessed to a free base for smoking. Causes euphoria and excess energy. Common health effects include heart attacks, respiratory failure, strokes, and seizures. Large amounts can cause bizarre and violent behavior. In rare cases, sudden death can occur on the first use of cocaine or unexpectedly thereafter.
Ecstacy	MDMA, XTC, X, Adam, hug, beans, love drug	A human-made drug that acts as both a stimulant and a hallucinogen. It is taken orally as a capsule or tablet. Short-term effects include feelings of mental stimu-lation, emotional warmth, enhanced sensory perception, and increased physical energy. Adverse health effects can include nausea, chills, sweating, teeth clenching, muscle cramping, and blurred vision.
Heroin	Smack, H, horse, ska, junk, and many others	An addictive drug that is processed from morphine and usually appears as a white or brown powder. Short-term effects include a surge of euphoria fol-lowed by intermittent wakefulness and

(continues)

Table 34-1   DRUGS OF ABUSE (CONTINUED)

NAME	STREET NAME	DRUG EFFECT
		drowsiness, with cloudy mental functioning. Associated with fatal overdose, particularly in users who inject. Known cases of transmission of HIV and hepatitis occurred from sharing needles. Long-term users may develop collapsed veins, heart and bloodstream infections, liver disease, and lung complications.
Inhalants	Whippets, snappers poppers,	Breathable, chemical vapors, often of household substances that are used for mind-altering effects. Most produce a rapid high that resembles alcohol intoxication. If a large amount is inhaled, many will cause anesthesia, a loss of sensation, and unconsciousness.
LSD	Acid, blotter, and many others	One of the strongest mood-altering drugs. It is used as tablets, capsules, liquid, or on absorbent paper. Causes unpredictable psychological effects. In large doses, users experience delusions and visual hallucinations. Physical effects include increased body temperature, heart rate, and blood pressure; sleeplessness; and loss of appetite.
Marijuana	Pot, ganga, weed, grass, and many others	The most commonly used illegal drug in the U.S. The main active chemical is THC. Usually smoked, but can be ingested in food. Short-term effects include memory and learning problems, distorted perception, and difficulty thinking and solving problems.
Methadone	Juice, meth (name also used for methamphetamine, below), amidone, chocolate chip cookies, fizzies, wafer	This is a prescription drug that is valued for treating heroin addiction and chronic pain. It has been abused by recreational drug users and is causing an alarming increase in overdoses and deaths. It does not produce a euphoria or rush, so users tend to take more to get the desired effect, with disastrous results. The drug has a long half life, so its effects are not always predictable to inexperienced users. It is available in tablet, liquid, or injectable preparations. Causes relaxation, pain relief, apathy, impaired judgment, sleepiness, impaired sense of reality. Physiologic effects include constricted pupils, slurred speech, nausea, respiratory depression, constipation. Overdoses are associated with respiratory depression, coma, and death.

Table 34-1   DRUGS OF ABUSE (CONTINUED)

NAME	STREET NAME	DRUG EFFECT
Methamphetamine	Speed, meth, chalk, ice, crystal, glass	A highly addictive man-made stimulant that is closely related to amphetamine, but has longer lasting and more toxic effects on the central nervous system. Ingredients vary depending on the recipe used to cook it, but can include lye and drain cleaner. It has a high potential for abuse and addiction. Increases wakefulness and physical activity and decreases appetite with weight loss. Chronic, long-term use can lead to psychotic behavior, paranoia, compulsive behavior, hallucinations, and stroke. Can be swallowed, inhaled, smoked, or injected.
PCP/ Phencyclidine	Angel dust, ozone, wack, rocket fuel, and many others	Illegally manufactured in labs and sold as tablets, capsules, or colored powder. It can be snorted, smoked, or eaten. It was originally developed in the 1950s as an IV anesthetic, but was never approved for human use because of problems during clinical studies, including intensely negative psychological effects. Many PCP users are brought to emergency rooms because of overdose or because of the drug's unpleasant psychological effects. In a hospital or detention setting, people high on PCP often become violent or suicidal.
Prescription drugs	Commonly abused drugs are those given for pain management, such as Oxycontin, Vicodin, Lortab, Codeine, Demerol, Dilaudid, Fentanyl, and others. Other drugs that are frequently abused include central nervous system depressants (prescribed to treat anxiety and sleep disorders), and stimulants (prescribed to treat narcolepsy, ADHD, and obesity).	Prescription drugs that are abused or used for nonmedical reasons can alter brain activity and lead to addiction. Long-term use of opioids or central nervous system depressants can lead to physical dependence and addiction. Taken in high doses, stimulants can lead to compulsive use, paranoia, dangerously high body temperatures, and irregular heartbeat.

Substance Withdrawal

Patients who are withdrawing from alcohol may have *delirium tremens (DTs)*. Withdrawal from other substances produces similar signs and symptoms. DTs are part of a serious withdrawal syndrome seen in persons who stop drinking alcohol following continuous and heavy consumption. They commonly begin 48 to 96 hours after taking the last drink. Signs and symptoms of DTs are:

• severe confusion

• tremors

• hallucinations

• overactivity of the nervous system

• seizures

• severe hypotension

DTs can become life threatening, and require immediate treatment. Inform the nurse promptly if a patient displays signs or symptoms of delirium tremens.

The substance abuser in withdrawal feels depressed and defensive. He or she needs to identify the stressors that bring on the need for alcohol or drugs and to find new ways of coping. This process takes professional skill, but you can:

• Not allow the substance abuser to manipulate you.

• Listen with empathy.

• Reflect the person's ideas and thoughts.

• Be sure alcohol and drugs are not available.

• Be consistent in the limits that have been set.

• Monitor for use of products such as mouthwash, which contains a large amount of alcohol and chemicals that may be used as inhalents. A substance abuser in withdrawal often turns to unlikely and/or dangerous items to relieve the symptoms of withdrawal.

MALADAPTIVE BEHAVIORS

Mental illness or maladaptive behavior occurs when behaviors and responses disrupt the person's ability to function smoothly within the family, environment, or community.

As a nursing assistant, you need to be aware that sometimes signs and symptoms such as fatigue, loss of appetite, insomnia, and pain may reflect either physical or emotional stress. Note and report any unusual behavior or symptoms. Be careful, however, to be objective. Do not make judgments about your findings.

CARING FOR THE BARIATRIC PATIENT

INTRODUCTION

Being *overweight* means having a body weight that is greater than is considered desirable or medically advisable. The definition of *obesity* varies, but it is usually considered being 20 to 30 percent above the ideal body weight. *Morbid obesity* is the term used to describe individuals who are 100 pounds or more over their ideal body weight.

Persons with obesity experience discrimination and prejudice in social and employment situations. Overweight people often feel deep emotional pain caused by the insensitivity of and stereotyping by the public at large. They may have limited access to public facilities. Obesity is a very misunderstood condition that has many causes. It adversely affects every body system, increases the risk for many other complications and diseases, and results in a shorter life span. Obesity places a great strain on the heart and lungs, and the extra weight of the chest makes breathing difficult. Persons with obesity often have relationship problems. Some have problems with mental disorders, while others are victims of physical and psychological abuse.

Comorbidities are diseases and medical conditions that are either caused by or contributed to by morbid obesity. They create risk factors and medical management problems, and increase the risks associated with weight loss surgery. Weight loss usually improves or eliminates many comorbid conditions. Sometimes comorbid conditions are so unstable that they must be treated before the patient can have weight loss surgery.

Bariatrics is a new field of medicine that focuses on the treatment and control of obesity, as well as the medical conditions and diseases associated with obesity. Bariatric patients have special medical needs, surgical needs, or both. Some hospitals and long-term care facilities have specialized units for care of bariatric patients.

WEIGHT AND BODY MASS INDEX

A person's *ideal body weight (IBW)* is determined by a mathematical formula. Ideal weight is a concept developed from life insurance statistics related to lifespan (longevity) and health. The registered dietitian routinely calculates the IBW for each patient. The formula he or she uses considers the person's height, age, sex, build, activity, medical condition, and need for nutrients. *Body mass index (BMI)* is also a consideration (Table 35-1). The BMI is a mathematical calculation used to determine whether a person is at a healthy, normal weight, is overweight, or obese. *Ideal weight* is considered as having a BMI that is less than 26. Obesity is a BMI of 30–39. Morbid obesity usually qualifies for surgical treatment, and means the

Table 35-1   BODY MASS INDEX TABLE

BMI Height (in inches)	19	20	21	22	23	24	25	26	27	28	29	30	31	32	33	34	35	36	37	38	39	40
																					Weight (in pounds)	
58	91	96	100	105	110	115	119	124	129	134	138	143	148	153	158	162	167	172	177	181	186	191
59	94	99	104	109	114	119	124	128	133	138	143	148	153	158	163	168	173	178	183	188	193	198
60	97	102	107	112	118	123	128	133	138	143	148	153	158	163	168	174	179	184	189	194	199	204
61	100	106	111	116	122	127	132	137	143	148	153	158	164	169	174	180	185	190	195	201	206	211
62	104	109	115	120	126	131	136	142	147	153	158	164	169	175	180	186	191	196	202	207	213	218
63	107	113	118	124	130	135	141	146	152	158	163	169	175	180	186	191	197	203	208	214	220	225
64	110	116	122	128	134	140	145	151	157	163	169	174	180	186	192	197	204	209	215	221	227	232
65	114	120	126	132	138	144	150	156	162	168	174	180	186	192	198	204	210	216	222	228	234	240
66	118	124	130	135	142	148	155	161	167	173	179	186	192	198	204	210	216	223	229	235	241	247
67	121	127	134	140	146	153	159	166	172	178	185	191	198	204	211	217	223	230	236	242	249	255
68	125	131	138	144	151	158	164	171	177	184	190	197	204	210	216	223	230	236	243	249	256	262
69	128	135	142	149	155	162	169	176	182	189	196	203	210	216	223	230	236	243	250	257	263	270
70	132	139	146	153	160	167	174	181	188	195	202	209	216	222	229	236	243	250	257	264	271	278
71	136	143	150	157	165	172	179	186	193	200	208	215	222	229	236	243	250	257	265	272	279	286
72	140	147	154	162	169	177	184	191	199	206	213	221	228	235	242	250	258	265	272	279	287	294
73	144	151	159	166	174	182	189	197	204	212	219	227	235	242	250	257	265	272	280	288	295	302
74	148	155	163	171	179	186	194	202	210	218	225	233	241	249	256	264	272	280	287	295	303	311
75	152	160	168	176	184	192	200	208	216	224	232	240	248	256	264	272	279	287	295	303	311	319
76	156	164	172	180	189	197	205	213	221	230	238	246	254	263	271	279	287	295	304	312	320	328

To use the table, find the appropriate height in the left-hand column labeled Height. Move across to a given weight. The number at the top of the column is the BMI at that height and weight. Pounds have been rounded off.

Table 35-2	CLASSIFICATION OF WEIGHT AND BODY MASS INDEX
BMI*	**CATEGORY**
<18.5	Underweight
18.5 to 24.99	Normal
25 to 26.9	Overweight
27 to 30	Mild obesity
31 to 35	Moderate obesity
36 to 40	Severe obesity
41 to 45	Morbid obesity
>50	Super obesity

person has a BMI of 40 or higher. Table 35-2 lists the categories for weight and body mass. This table is used when determining whether a patient is a candidate for weight loss surgery.

ENVIRONMENTAL MODIFICATIONS

Many hospitals admit bariatric patients to private rooms that have been modified to meet their needs. The private room upholds the patient's dignity, and prevents potential infringement on the rights of other patients. The room should be equipped with:
• wide doorways
• a floor-mounted toilet
• one or more fans
• a bed that will support the patient's weight that is spacious enough to enable him or her to move freely
• a chair that is about the size of a loveseat

Optional equipment and supplies that may also be needed include:
• a wide wheelchair
• a wide walker
• an overbed trapeze

• a scale that will weigh patients who weigh more than 350 pounds
• pressure-reducing overlays to fit the bed and wheelchair
• a ceiling or floor mounted electrical or mechanical lift that can safely be used for patients weighing more than 300 pounds; slings for the lift must also be wide enough and sturdy enough for bariatric patients
• extra large or ample size gowns large enough to fit bariatric patients
• thigh cuffs, extra-large blood pressure cuffs, or another means of measuring the patients' blood pressure

PATIENT CARE

Care that is routine for normal-size patients presents unique challenges in the bariatric population. The patients will be more time consuming than many of the others you care for. The nurse will adjust your assignment to allow time to provide conscientious patient care. Routine ADL care given by nursing assistants often needs procedural modifications for these patients. Some activities of daily living are difficult for the patients to do. They often feel guilty when they are admitted to the hospital, because they know that their size makes it hard for staff to care for them.

Skin Care

The skin is the largest organ of the body, and the bariatric patient has much extra skin. Usually, it has been stretched and is easily injured. The bariatric patient's skin is usually very tender, as well as sensitive to the effects of moisture, pressure, friction, and sheer force. The patient is at very high risk for pressure ulcers. Bariatric patients have many skin folds. Most patients have a fatty apron of abdominal skin called the *panniculus* or *pannus*. (A pannus is a hanging flap of skin.) The patient's skin must be kept very clean and dry to reduce the risk of complications.

The areas between the skin folds are warm, moist, and dark, creating perfect conditions for the proliferation of pathogens. Monitor the skin folds frequently to make sure they are not red or weeping in appearance. Wash and dry the skin folds frequently. Excessive moisture from perspiration in the warm, moist, dark environment presents a great risk for a painful yeast infection called *intertrigo, candidiasis,* or *moniliasis.* Make sure the areas between the skin folds are kept dry. If necessary, a flannel bath blanket can be cut and folded to place in the skin folds. A better alternative is to obtain a supply of flannel receiving blankets, such as those used in the newborn nursery, and fold and place them between the skin folds. Avoid the temptation to use washcloths and towels in these fragile skin areas. The rough surface texture will further irritate tender skin.

If the patient is unconscious or using ventilator support, make sure to carefully check the skin folds behind the neck. These tend to become wet from sputum and saliva, and the patient's position produces constant pressure, placing him or her at risk of both yeast infection and pressure ulcers. The increased body weight promotes rapid ulcer development. Reposition the head manually each time the patient is turned. Otherwise, it tends to stay in the same position, and a pressure ulcer will develop quickly. Make sure that the various lines and tubes are not tunneled into, trapped between, or pressing on the patient's skin. Elevate the heels off the surface of the bed, or use a bariatric product that relieves pressure on the heel.

BARIATRIC SURGERY

Bariatric surgery is surgery on the stomach and/or intestines to help the patient with morbid or super obesity lose weight. Different procedures may be done, depending on patient needs and doctor preference. Surgical treatment is usually reserved for persons with a body mass index over 40. It is sometimes used as a treatment for people with a BMI between 35 and 40 who have health problems and potentially serious co-morbidities, such as heart disease or type 2 diabetes.

Postoperative Care

Routine postoperative care given on the evening after surgery will probably include remote telemetry monitoring. The patient may be using oxygen through a cannula. Nursing assistants may be responsible for numerous procedures.

- Vital signs according to postoperative routine, then hourly or as instructed by the nurse

- Abdominal binder
- Ice packs to the incision
- Check dressing over incision and drain hourly, or as instructed
- Use the incentive spirometer at least 10 times every hour
- Coughing and deep breathing
- Antiembolism hosiery, circulation checks to feet every 2 to 4 hours
- Sequential compression devices may be ordered
- Up in chair with assistance one or more times

- Catheter care
- Patient is NPO except for ice chips
- Intake and output monitoring and recording
- Monitor the pulse oximeter for alarms

The patient's activities and diet will be increased gradually, as tolerated. If no complications are present, he or she is discharged on postoperative day 3. The health care provider, surgeon, and dietitian will continue to follow the patient's progress for a year after surgery.

DEATH AND DYING

36

As a nursing assistant, you will be providing care throughout the period of dying and into the after-death (postmortem) period. Accepting the idea that death is the natural result of the life process may help you respond to your patient's needs more generously.

You must accept the patient's behavior with understanding (see Table 36-1), interpret the patient's very real need for family support, and support the family members in meeting their own needs during this adjustment period.

Table 36-1 EMOTIONAL RESPONSES TO DYING

STAGES OF GRIEF	RESPONSE OF THE NURSING ASSISTANT
Denial	Reflect patient's statements, but try not to confirm or deny the fact that the patient is dying. Example: *"The lab tests can't be right—I don't have cancer."* *"It must have been difficult for you to learn the results of your tests."*
Anger	Understand the source of the patient's anger. Provide understanding and support. Listen. Try to meet reasonable needs and demands quickly. Example: *"This food is terrible—not fit to eat."* *"Let me see if I can find something that would appeal to you more."*
Bargaining	If it is possible to meet the patient's requests, do so. Listen attentively. Example: *"If only God will spare me this, I'll go to church every week."* *"Would you like a visit from your clergyperson?"*
Depression	Avoid clichés that dismiss the patient's depression ("It could be worse—you could be in more pain"). Be caring and supportive. Let the patient know that it is all right to be depressed. Example: *"There just isn't any sense in going on."* *"I understand you are feeling very depressed."*
Acceptance	Do not assume that, because the patient has accepted death, she or he is unafraid or does not need emotional support. Listen attentively and be supportive and caring. Example: *"I feel so alone."* *"I am here with you. Would you like to talk?"*

SUPPORTIVE CARE

Supportive care means that the patient's life will not be artificially prolonged but that the patient will be kept comfortable physically, mentally, and emotionally. Supportive care includes:

- Oxygen to ease breathing if the patient needs it
- Food and fluids that the patient can consume by mouth
- Medications for pain, nausea, anxiety, or other physical or emotional discomforts
- The continuation of physical care such as grooming and hygiene, cleanliness, positioning, and range-of-motion exercises
- Caring and emotional support of staff

LIFE-SUSTAINING TREATMENT

All patients deserve supportive care, but for terminally or critically ill patients, supportive care means the absence of life-sustaining treatment. Life-sustaining treatment means giving medications and treatments for the purpose of maintaining life. It includes:

- Being placed on a ventilator to maintain breathing
- Receiving cardiopulmonary resuscitation (CPR) if cardiac arrest occurs (the heart and lungs stop functioning)
- Artificial nutrition through a feeding tube or hyperalimentation device
- Blood transfusions
- Surgery
- Radiation therapy
- Chemotherapy
- Other treatments that will maintain life

Note: Radiation therapy and chemotherapy may also be given to relieve pain, not to extend life.

YOUR RESPONSIBILITY

As a nursing assistant, you must be aware of the patient's status for supportive care or life-sustaining treatment. The person on supportive care will have a no-code order or DNR (do not resuscitate) order. This means that no extraordinary means, such as CPR to resuscitate the person, will be used to prevent death.

Witnessing Advance Directives

The nursing assistant must become familiar with facility policies and state laws for witnessing advance directives. In many states, persons who care for the patient are not permitted to witness advance directives. In most states, caregivers cannot be legally appointed to be the medical decision maker for a patient unless they are related by blood or marriage.

Withdrawing or Modifying Advance Directives

Patients may withdraw or modify their advance directives at any time. If a patient informs you of changes that affect the advance directive, notify the nurse promptly.

THE ROLE OF THE NURSING ASSISTANT

As a nursing assistant, you spend much time with the patient, and you have a unique opportunity to be a source of strength and comfort. You must behave in a way that instills confidence in both the patient and the patient's family. There are some things to keep in mind:

- Your response should be consistent. It should be guided by the patient's attitude and the care plan.
- You must be open and receptive, because the terminal patient's attitude may change from day to day.

- Make sure you inform the nurse of incidents related to the patient that reflect moods and needs.
- Remember, each person's idea of death and the hereafter differs. You must be open to patients' ideas and not force your own upon them.
- Your own feelings about death and dying influence your ability to care for the dying patient. Honestly explore your feelings by talking about them with others until you can resolve any conflicts you may have. Your acceptance of death as a natural occurrence will enable you to meet patient needs in a realistic manner.
- Give your best and most careful nursing care, with special attention to comfort measures such as mouth care and fluid intake.
- You should be quietly empathetic and carry out your duties in a calm, efficient way.

PROVIDING FOR SPIRITUAL NEEDS

Many people find spiritual faith to be a source of great comfort during difficult times. Refer to Table 36-2.

Be aware that dying is a lonely business, a journey each person must finish alone. Until the final moment comes, privacy, but not total solitude, should be the guiding rule.

FAMILY NEEDS

It is important to remember the family and other loved ones when a patient is dying. Check the policies of your health care facility and assist in the following actions:

- Allow the family to be with the patient as they desire.
- Allow the family to assist with some of the care, if they wish to do so; for example, moistening the patient's lips or giving a backrub.

- Inform the family where they can get a cup of coffee or a meal.
- Show the family where they can use a telephone in private.
- If a family member stays during the night, offer a pillow and blanket. Some facilities provide recliners or cots for family members.
- Avoid being judgmental of family members. Remember that each person grieves in his or her own way. The emotions that others see are not necessarily an accurate indication of what the individual is feeling.

PHYSICAL CHANGES AS DEATH APPROACHES

As death approaches, there are notable physical changes. As these changes occur, report them immediately to the nurse.

- The patient becomes less responsive.
- Body functions slow down.
- The patient loses voluntary and involuntary muscle control.
- The patient may involuntarily void and defecate.
- The jaw tends to drop.
- Breathing becomes irregular and shallow.
- Circulation slows, and the extremities become cold. The pulse becomes rapid and progressively weaker.
- Skin pales.
- The eyes stare and do not respond to light.
- Hearing seems to be the last sense to be lost. Do not assume that because death is approaching, the patient can no longer hear. You must be careful what you say.

As it becomes clear that death will occur very soon, you should call the nurse, who will supervise the care during the final moments of life.

Table 36-2 BELIEFS AND PRACTICES RELATED TO DYING AND DEATH FOR MAJOR RELIGIONS

RELIGION	AUTOPSY	ORGAN DONATION	BELIEFS AND PRACTICES
Judaism (Orthodox)	Only in special circumstances	With consultation of a rabbi	Visits to the dying are a religious duty.
			Witness must be present if death occurs, to protect family and commit soul to God.
			Torah and Psalms may be read and prayers recited.
			Conversation is kept to a minimum.
			Someone should be with the body after death until burial, usually within 24 hours.
			Body must not be touched 8 to 30 minutes after death.
			Medical personnel should not touch or wash body unless death occurs on Jewish Sabbath; then care may be given by staff wearing gloves.
			Water is removed from the room.
			Mirrors may be covered at family's request.
			Jewish practices and beliefs can be very different from family to family. Asking the patient or family members about their practices is probably best.
Hinduism	Permitted	Permitted	Priest ties thread around neck or wrist of deceased and pours water in the mouth.
			Only family and friends touch body.

(continues)

235

Table 36-2 BELIEFS AND PRACTICES RELATED TO DYING AND DEATH FOR MAJOR RELIGIONS (CONTINUED)

RELIGION	AUTOPSY	ORGAN DONATION	BELIEFS AND PRACTICES
Buddhism	Personal preference	Permitted	Buddhist priest is present at death. Last rites are chanted at the bedside.
Islam (Muslim)	Only for medical or legal reasons	Not permitted	Before death, read Koran and pray. Patient confesses sins and asks forgiveness of family. Only family touches or washes body. After death, turn head towards right shoulder.
Roman Catholic	Permitted	Permitted	Sacrament of the Sick administered to ill patients, to patients in imminent danger, or shortly after death.
Christian Scientist	Unlikely	Not permitted	No ritual is performed before or after death.
Church of Christ	Permitted	Permitted	No ritual is performed before or after death.
Jehovah's Witness	Only if required by law	Not permitted	No ritual is performed before or after death.
Baptist	Permitted	Permitted	Clergy ministers through counseling and prayers.
Episcopalian	Permitted	Permitted	Last rites are optional.
Lutheran	Permitted	Permitted	Last rites are optional.
Eastern Orthodox Christian	Not encouraged	Not encouraged	Last rites are mandatory and are given by ordained priest.

SIGNS OF DEATH

After death, changes continue to take place in the body. These are called moribund changes.

- Pupils become permanently dilated.
- There is no pulse or respiration.
- Heat is gradually lost from the body.
- The patient may urinate, defecate, or release flatus.
- Blood pools in the lowest areas of the body, giving a purplish discoloration to those areas.
- Within 2 to 4 hours, body rigidity, called rigor mortis, develops.
- Unless the body is embalmed within 24 hours, there is indication of progressive protein breakdown.

POSTMORTEM CARE

The patient's body should be treated with respect at all times. Before death occurs, the limbs should be straightened and the head elevated on a pillow. The body should be cleaned by gently washing it with warm water. Discharges must be washed off and wiped away.

Care of the body after death is called postmortem care. This may be your responsibility. You may find it easier if you ask a coworker to assist.

- Use gloves when giving postmortem care. The body may continue to be infectious following death.
- Treat the body with the same dignity you would a living person.
- Some facilities prefer to have the patient left alone until the mortuary staff arrive. Your responsibility will be only to prepare the body for viewing by the family.
- Check the procedure manual for a list of supplies used for postmortem care (Figure 36.1).

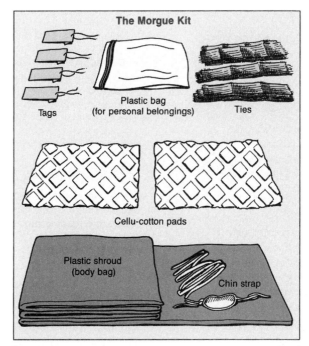

The Morgue Kit

Tags

Plastic bag
(for personal belongings)

Ties

Cellu-cotton pads

Plastic shroud
(body bag)

Chin strap

Figure 36-1 Supplies for postmortem care. These are usually found in a morgue pack or morgue kit. Some facilities do not use these items. Follow your facility policies for preparing the body.

CARE OF THE ELDERLY AND CHRONICALLY ILL

CHAPTER

37

PHYSICAL CHANGES IN AGING

Refer to Table 37-1.

EMOTIONAL ADJUSTMENTS TO AGING

Frustration is an emotion frequently experienced by the elderly—frustration at physical limitations and at having less control over their own lives. That is why it is important to allow them the opportunity to make as many decisions as possible.

NUTRITIONAL NEEDS

Residents who are at greatest risk of malnutrition and unintentional weight loss are those who:

- Need help eating and drinking
- Eat less than half their meals and/or planned snacks
- Have mouth pain
- Have no dentures or have dentures that do not fit correctly
- Have difficulty chewing or swallowing
- Have difficulty getting utensils or glasses to their mouth
- Cough or choke while eating
- Are sad, have crying spells, or withdraw from others
- Are confused, wander, or pace
- Have diabetes, lung disease, cancer, HIV, or other chronic diseases

Because of loss of muscle tone, three intestinal problems are commonly seen. They are:

- Constipation—difficulty in eliminating sold waste
- Flatulence—gas production
- Diverticulosis—small pockets (diverticula) of weakened intestinal wall

Residents Receiving Tube Feedings

Tube feedings are common treatments in the long-term care facility. Residents receiving tube feedings are also at nutritional risk. Their medical needs sometimes change, and tube feeding formula and fluid orders must be adjusted to keep up with their body's demands. Signs and symptoms that a resident is at risk for experiencing tube feeding complications are:

- Nausea
- Vomiting
- Diarrhea
- Swollen stomach
- Constipation
- Excessive flatus, cramping
- Pain, redness, heat, swelling, crusting, or fluid oozing from the site where the feeding tube enters the body
- Cough
- Wet breathing
- Feeling that something is caught in the throat
- Complaints of dryness or discomfort in the mouth or throat
- Pulling at or removing the feeding tube

Table 37-1   PHYSICAL CHANGES OF AGING

BODY SYSTEM	PHYSICAL CHANGES
Integumentary	• Hair loses color and becomes thinner. • Skin dries, becomes less elastic; wrinkles develop. • Skin is fragile and tears easily. • Bruises easily (senile purpura common). • Reduced blood flow in vessels that nourish the skin results in delayed healing. • Fingernails and toenails thicken. • Sweat glands do not excrete perspiration as readily. • Oil glands do not secrete as much oil. • There is increased sensitivity to cold. • Skin discolorations (age spots) become more common. • Blood supply to the feet and legs is reduced, increasing risk of injury and ulcers, feeling of coldness.
Nervous	• Tasks involving speed, balance, coordination, and fine motor activities take longer because of slowed transmission of nerve impulses. • Balance and coordination problems as a result of deterioration in the nerve terminals that provide information to the brain about body movement and position. • Temperature regulation is less effective. • Deep sleep is shortened, more awakenings during the night. • Brain cells are lost, but intelligence remains intact unless disease is present. • Decreased sensitivity of nerve receptors in skin (heat, cold, pain, pressure). • Risk of injury increases because of decreased ability to feel pressure and temperature changes. • Decreased blood flow to the brain, which may result in mental confusion and memory loss.
Sensory	• More difficult to see close objects. • Night vision may decrease. • Cataracts (clouding of the lens of the eye) are more common. • Dryness and itching of the eyes as a result of decreased secretion of fluids. • Side vision and depth perception diminish. • Hearing diminishes in many elderly persons. • Smell receptors and taste buds are less sensitive, so foods have less taste.

(continues)

Table 37-1 PHYSICAL CHANGES OF AGING (CONTINUED)

BODY SYSTEM	PHYSICAL CHANGES
Musculoskeletal	• Loss of elasticity of muscles and decrease in size of muscle mass resulting in reduced strength, flexibility, endurance, muscle tone, and delayed reaction time. • Slower movements. • Bones lose minerals, become brittle, and break more easily; arthritis and osteoporosis common. • Spine becomes less stable and flexible, increasing the risk of injury. • Posture may become slumped over because of weakness in back muscles. • Degenerative changes in the joints result in limited movement, stiffness, and pain.
Respiratory	• Lung capacity decreases as a result of muscular rigidity in the lungs. • The ability to cough is less effective; results in pooling of secretions and fluid in the lungs, increasing the risk of infection and choking. • Shortness of breath on exertion as a result of aging changes in lungs. • Gas exchange in the lungs is less effective, resulting in decreased oxygenation.
Urinary	• Kidneys decrease in size. • Urine production is less efficient. • Bladder capacity decreases, increasing the frequency of urination. • Kidney function increases at rest, causing increased urination at night. • Weakening of bladder muscles, causing leaking of urine or inability to empty the bladder completely; complete emptying of bladder becomes more difficult. • Enlargement of the prostate gland in the male, causing increased frequency of urination, dribbling, urinary obstruction, and urinary retention.
Digestive	• Decreased saliva production in the mouth, causing difficulty with swallowing, digestion of starches, and increased risk for tooth decay. • Taste buds on the tongue decrease, beginning with sweet and salt; changes in taste buds may result in appetite changes and increase in condiment use. • Gag reflex is less effective, increasing the risk of choking. • Movement of food into the stomach through the esophagus is slower. • Slower digestion of food in the stomach, so food remains there longer before moving to the small intestine.

Table 37-1   PHYSICAL CHANGES OF AGING (CONTINUED)

BODY SYSTEM	PHYSICAL CHANGES
	• Flatulence increases. • Indigestion and slower absorption of fat as a result of decreased digestive enzymes. • Food movement through the large intestine is slower, resulting in constipation.
Cardiovascular	• Heart rate slows, causing a slower pulse and less efficient circulation. This results in decreased energy and a slower response, causing the individual to tire easily. • Blood vessels lose elasticity and develop calcium deposits, causing vessels to narrow. • Blood pressure increases because of changes to the blood vessel walls. • Heart rate takes longer to return to normal after exercise. • Veins enlarge, causing blood vessels close to the skin surface to become more prominent. • Heart may not pump as efficiently, leading to decreased cardiac output and circulation.
Endocrine	• Decrease in levels of estrogen, progesterone. • Hot flashes, nervous feelings. • Higher levels of parathormone and thyroid-stimulating hormone. • Delayed release of insulin, increasing blood sugar level; incidence of diabetes increases greatly with age. • Metabolism rate and body function slow, reducing the amount of calories needed for the body to function normally. This increases the risk of overweight and obesity.
Reproductive	*Females:* • Fewer female hormones are produced. • Ovulation and menstrual cycle cease. • Vaginal walls are thinner and drier. • Vagina becomes shorter and narrower. • Breast tissue decreases, and the muscles supporting the breasts weaken. *Males:* • Scrotum is less firm. • Prostate gland may enlarge. • Hormone production decreases, decreasing the size of testes and lowering sperm count. • More time is required for an erection.

Nursing Assistant Actions

Nursing assistant actions to take when residents are at risk of tube feeding complications are:

- Keep the head of the bed elevated 30 to 45 degrees any time the tube feeding is running and for 1 hour after feeding is completed.
- Provide frequent oral care.
- Follow the nurse's instructions and care plan for care of the skin around the feeding tube.
- Move the resident carefully and position to avoid tension or traction on the tube.
- Make sure that the tube is not kinked or obstructed.
- Give the resident something to hold if he or she is pulling on the feeding tube; notify the nurse promptly.
- Turn the resident on the side if coughing or choking.
- Report observations and warning signs to the nurse promptly.

HYDRATION NEEDS

Like malnutrition, dehydration can and does occur in long-term care residents. This is partly due to decreased thirst in the elderly. Some residents avoid fluids because they fear incontinence. Some residents do not like to drink water but willingly accept other liquids. The majority of residents who become dehydrated do so because of medical illness and the physical or mental inability to ask for liquids, hold the cup, pour from the pitcher, or drink from a straw without assistance. Extra fluid is needed in all residents in very hot weather. Dehydration can be a very serious condition in the elderly, causing delirium and other complications. Residents who are becoming dehydrated or are at high risk for dehydration are those who:

- Drink fewer than 6 cups of liquid a day

- Have dry mouth
- Have cracked lips
- Have sunken eyes
- Have dark urine
- Need help drinking from a glass
- Have trouble swallowing liquids
- Have diarrhea, vomiting, or fever
- Are mentally confused
- Are weak or tired
- Are lethargic and have difficulty staying awake

Nursing Assistant Actions

Nursing assistant actions to prevent dehydration are:

- Offering the resident a drink each time you enter the room; set a goal, such as 2 to 4 ounces of liquid each time
- Drinking with the resident, if permitted
- Providing fluids the resident likes, as permitted on the diet
- Making sure fresh water is available, that the resident can reach it, and the pitcher and cup are light enough to hold
- Providing physical assistance to pour and consume fluids, as needed
- Offering ice chips, if permitted
- Following all swallowing precautions listed on the care plan
- Alternating liquids with solids when feeding meals
- Encouraging the resident to attend activities involving food and fluids
- Accurately monitoring and recording intake and output, when ordered
- Promptly notifying the nurse of your observations

PREVENTING INFECTIONS IN RESIDENTS

The elderly do not readily show signs of infection. This means they may be sick for some time before you recognize the problem.

- The elderly do not always develop a fever with an infection. The average temperature for an older person may be a degree or two lower than that of a younger person. Therefore, average temperature may represent an increase or fever.

The elderly are also more likely to develop serious complications from infections. A simple urinary tract infection can result in bacteremia (blood infection), causing the resident to become acutely ill. Sepsis (presence of pus-forming and other pathogens or their toxins in the blood) is also a serious complication of infection in the elderly. These conditions can be fatal to a person who has little ability to cope with additional health problems.

Rather than developing a fever, residents with sepsis often become hypothermic. Monitor residents with abnormally low body temperature closely, and notify the nurse promptly of an *abnormally low* body temperature in an elderly person.

Nursing Assistant Actions

Prevention of infection in residents is an ongoing concern. You can take the following steps to help in this process:

- Assist residents to maintain an adequate fluid intake.
- Assist residents to maintain adequate nutritional intake.
- Report to the nurse when residents eat less or refuse food.
- Assist residents to perform exercise programs established by the nurse or physical therapist.
- Follow positioning schedules and orders for range-of-motion exercises and ambulation.
- Attend to residents' personal hygiene and grooming needs.

- Inspect the body and mouth when performing these procedures.
- Toilet residents regularly who need assistance. Some residents hesitate to drink fluids for fear that they will be incontinent.
- When caring for incontinent residents, be sure to wipe female residents using strokes from front to back.
- Perform catheter care as directed.
- Avoid opening the closed drainage system.
- Use aseptic technique when emptying the catheter bag.
- Observe residents carefully and report any unusual signs or changes. Urinary tract infections may be discovered from changes in the urine or by incontinence.
- The first sign of any infection is disorientation in people who are not usually disoriented.
- A change in behavior may indicate an infection.
- Incidents of falling often occur in residents with infections.

DELIRIUM

Delirium is an acute confusional state caused by reversible medical problems. It is common in the elderly, particularly those over age 75. Delirium is a nonspecific symptom of acute illness and dehydration in the elderly. It is a very serious condition. If delirium is unrecognized and untreated, the mortality rate is high, particularly in residents with chronic disease, mental problems, or dementia.

Signs and Symptoms of Delirium

Delirium develops rapidly, often within a few hours or days. Delirium may not be recognized until the resident is critically ill.

Any change in a resident's mental status is significant.

Residents with acute delirium develop disorientation, behavioral changes, and decreased awareness of the environment. Other common signs and symptoms are:

- Reduced or fluctuating levels of consciousness
- Misinterpreting the environment, misunderstanding or misinterpreting conversations
- Hallucinations
- Illusions
- Delusions
- Insomnia and disturbance of sleep-wake cycle
- Change in motor activity
- Mental confusion and memory impairment

Nursing Assistant Responsibilities

Early identification and careful observation are essential to preventing more serious problems. As a nursing assistant, you will work more closely with residents than other caregivers. You will become familiar with the resident's usual or normal condition. If something differs from the resident's usual condition, do not overlook it.

KEEPING RESIDENTS SAFE

Prevention of Falls

The environment can be altered to meet the needs of elderly persons:

- Noise increases disorientation and can create anxiety even in alert persons. This increases the risk of falls. Minimizing all noises reduces this risk.
- All tubs and showers should have chairs so residents can remain

seated throughout the procedure. Lifts for tubs avoid the need for the resident to stand in the tub. Avoid using oils that can make the tub bottom slippery.

- Check residents' clothing for fit. Loose shoes and laces, slippers, long robes, and slacks increase the risk of falling.
- Observe ambulatory residents when they get out of bed and chairs, when they get off the toilet, and when they walk.
  - Give instructions to residents who have unsafe habits.
  - When you help dependent residents transfer, always use the method indicated in the care plan.
- Side rails are a frequent cause of falls. In some situations, half rails are more effective. Follow the care plan.

CARING FOR RESIDENTS WITH DEMENTIA

Dementia is not a disease but is a group of symptoms seen in a number of different diseases (Table 37-2). Alzheimer's disease is the most common form of dementia.

Goals of Care

When you are caring for residents with dementia, remember to:

- Protect residents from physical injury.
- Allow residents to maintain independence as long as possible.
- Provide physical and mental activities within residents' abilities.
- Support residents' dignity and self-esteem.

To meet these goals, the care must be:

- Consistent

Table 37-2   DESCRIPTION OF MAJOR FORMS OF DEMENTIA

DISEASE	FEATURES	COURSE
Alzheimer's disease	Lack of chemical in brain, causing neuro-fibrillary tangles, neuritic plaques	Onset age: 60–80 Slowly progressive
Multi-infarct dementia	Interference with blood circulation in brain cells due to arteriosclerosis or atherosclerosis	Onset age: 55–70 Outcome depends on rate of damage to brain cells
Huntington's disease	Inherited from either parent who has gene for the disease	Onset age: 25–45 Average duration 15 years
Parkinson's disease	Deficiency of chemical in brain (dopamine)	Onset age: 55–60 Several years' duration
Creutzfeldt-Jakob disease	Noninflammatory virus causes changes in brain	Onset age: usually 50–60 Rapidly progressive
Syphilis	Spirochete (bacteria) causes brain damage	Occurs 15–20 years after primary infection
AIDS dementia	HIV-1 infection	Symptoms sometimes pre-cede diagnosis of AIDS

- Provided with a structured but flexible routine

- Given in a peaceful, quiet environment that is simple, uncluttered, and unchanged

Managing Behavior Problems

- Remember that when the ability to use speech is lost, communication occurs through nonverbal means:
  - Biting, scratching, and kicking may be the only way the resident can express displeasure.
  - Watch for facial expressions and body language for clues to feelings and moods.
  - Learn what triggers agitation or anger. Work on preventing these situations.

- Use techniques of diversion and distraction.

- Realize that people with dementia are not responsible for what they do or say:
  - Their behavior is not intentional, and they cannot change.
  - They are not aware of what they are doing.
  - They lose the ability to control their impulses.
  - Avoid confrontations and always allow them to "save face"—that is, keep their dignity.
  - No one really knows what is happening in the minds of people with dementia.

- Modify your behavior in response to the person's behavior.

SPECIAL PROBLEMS

Wandering and Pacing

Nursing Assistant Approaches
- Allow the resident to wander.
- Avoid restraints, if possible.
- Walk with the resident, whenever possible.
- Adapt the environment to the wandering resident, to ensure it is safe and secure.
- Keep the resident's stress as low as possible.
- Try to meet the resident's needs for hunger, thirst, and elimination.
- Approach the resident in a calm, nonthreatening manner.
- Avoid forcing your own agenda on the resident.
- Use gentle persuasion. Avoid making too many demands on the resident during activities of daily living (ADLs) and direct care.
- Keep instructions simple and brief.
- As the resident completes one task, give him or her another.
- Be patient, calm, and reassuring.
- Compliment the resident for his or her successes, even if they are small.

Other approaches that may be effective:
- Taking the resident to the bathroom frequently.
- Adjusting the room temperature and ensuring the resident is wearing appropriate clothing for the temperature and season.
- Reducing environmental noise and stimulation; check residents' yelling, television, intercom announcements, and other sources of noise in the facility.
- Providing something to eat or drink.
- Informing the nurse if the resident complains of pain; he or she may not admit to having "pain" but may admit to having pressure, discomfort, or another unpleasant sensation.
- Providing a magazine, newspaper, book, or picture album.
- Visiting with the resident.
- Escorting the resident to activities.
- Having the resident fold towels and washcloths, perform a repetitious task, or sort other harmless items.
- Providing a stereo with earphones and playing soft, soothing music or the resident's favorite type of music, if known. This approach is often effective when others fail.
- Placing an identifying object, such as a bow, hat, or gender-appropriate decoration on the door of the resident's room and directing him or her to it.
- Making sure the resident wears glasses and hearing aid, as appropriate. Wandering may worsen if the resident misinterprets environmental signals.
- Avoiding clutter and safety hazards in the environment.
- Ensuring that chemicals and potential hazards are stored properly.
- Providing a night light at night or leaving the bathroom light on.
- If nighttime wandering is a problem, avoiding naps during the day. Limit caffeinated food and beverages.
- Avoiding the use of side rails. The resident may climb the rails, resulting in a serious fall.
- Attaching the call signal cord to the resident's clothing so the cord will pull from the wall and turn the signal on when he or she rises. Other types of tab signals or magnetic sensor systems may be used to alert staff if the resident rises or attempts to leave the facility through an exit door.
- Avoiding restraints, which often worsen agitation.
- Always knowing what the resident is wearing. Write this information

down at the beginning and end of each shift.

Agitation, Anxiety, and Catastrophic Reactions

Nursing Assistant Approaches

Agitation and anxiety are shown by an increase in physical activity, such as pacing. If appropriate interventions are not implemented in time, a catastrophic reaction will likely occur. You may note any or all of the following:
- Increased physical activity
- Increased talking or mumbling
- Explosive behavior with physical violence

To avoid catastrophic reactions:
- Monitor behavior closely.
- Watch for signs of increasing agitation.
- Check to see if the resident:
  - Is hungry.
  - Needs to go to the bathroom.
  - Is too hot or too cold.
  - Is overtired or in pain.
  - Has signs of physical illness.
- Check the environment for:
  - Too much noise.
  - Too many people.
  - Staff anxiety.
  - Television programs. People with dementia cannot distinguish fantasy from reality.
- Avoid forcing the resident to make decisions.

When agitation or catastrophic reactions occur:
- Do not use physical restraints or force in any attempt to subdue the resident. This increases agitation and can result in injury to the resident or staff.
- Avoid having several staff persons approach the resident at the same time. This is frightening to the resident.
- Use a soft, calm voice.
- Do not try to reason with the resident.
- Using touch may or may not be appropriate.

Sundowning

Nursing Assistant Approaches

Sundowning means that the resident has increased confusion during the late afternoon, evening, or night. It is sometimes prevented by avoiding too much activity before bedtime and by establishing a consistent bedtime routine.
- Overfatigue can cause sundowning.
- Encourage the resident to nap or rest in the early afternoon.
- Try to prevent the resident from sleeping too much during the day.
- The evening meal should be eaten at least 2 hours before bedtime.
- Eliminate or reduce caffeine from the resident's diet.
- Involve the resident in quiet evening activities, soft music, or interactions with a caregiver or family member.
- Provide a light bedtime snack that is easily chewed and digested.
- Take the resident to the bathroom.
- Allow sufficient time for bladder and bowel elimination.
- Give a slow back massage.
- Check with family members and continue the resident's established habits, such as wearing socks to bed, using two pillows, or having a night light.
- Check the lighting of the room. Shadows and reflections are disturbing.
- If the resident awakens during the night, repeat the bedtime routine. If this is ineffective and the resident does not remain in bed, try a recliner or Alzheimer's chair.

HOME CARE

The nurse discusses the plans with the client and then develops the assignment for the nursing assistant. You may be assigned to care for several clients or a particular client for:

- A specified number of hours daily
- A specified period 2 or 3 days per week
- A long-term period
- A brief period

Guidelines for Avoiding Liability

- Be sure you are given a job description upon employment that lists your specific duties and responsibilities. In some areas, home health aides are only allowed to do certain assigned tasks when working with an insurance company or Medicare. Auditors check the tasks assigned and confirm what is actually done in the client's home.
- Carry out procedures carefully and do them as you were taught.
- Always keep safety factors in mind and be on the lookout for possible hazards.
- Be familiar with the client's rights.
- Ask for assistance if you are assigned to a procedure that you have never performed before.

Make sure the procedure is within the legal boundaries of nursing assistant practice.

- Do only those tasks that are assigned to you.

- Know how to contact the supervising nurse for questions and issues related to the care of your client. Do not overstep your authority.
- Know how and when to contact emergency services for the client.
- Document your care and observations carefully and completely.
- Participate in care conferences with the other team members.

RECORD KEEPING

Two types of records are compiled by the nursing assistant giving home care. They are time/travel records and client care records.

Time/travel records are a record of how you spend your time in the client's home. Fill in the record as you complete each assignment. Do not wait until the end of the day or your assigned time and then try to rely on your memory.

Client care records are a record of:
- Care given, such as bathing, positioning, range-of-motion exercises
- Client's responses to care
- Housekeeping tasks completed, if assigned to you by the nurse
- Observations:
  - Condition of skin
  - Vital signs
  - Elimination; bowel and urine
  - Food and fluid intake
  - Appetite
  - Incidents such as client falls
  - Any observation that indicates a change in the client's health status

– Mental status: orientation, alertness, mood, and behavior

THE NURSING BAG

Most home health care workers carry a nursing bag stocked with the supplies they use routinely in client care. Carry enough supplies so you do not have to replenish it during a shift. Use a tote bag, back pack, or carrying case that keeps supplies organized and easy to find. The fabric or outside of the bag should be washable or easy to clean. Clean and restock your bag daily. Bring it into your house at night or leave it in the clinical office. Never leave it in the car. This invites theft, and heat and cold extremes may damage some supplies. People see the bag and associate it with helping clients, so make it clear that the bag does not contain any medications or syringes. Store the bag out of sight and lock the doors when you are not in the car.

Nursing Bag Supplies

Customize your nursing bag to include items that are necessary and convenient. Your agency may have a basic supply list. If not, consider your responsibilities and assignments, and pack a basic list of supplies to get started, such as those listed in Table 38-1.

Place your nursing bag on a barrier, such as a piece of newspaper, waxed paper, or a blue pad in the client's home. When leaving, discard trash, including the barrier pad, into a plastic bag and tie the top closed.

Table 38-1 SUGGESTED NURSING BAG SUPPLIES	
• Cell phone • Phone numbers • Pens • Paper or memo book • Extra forms for documentation • Waterless (alcohol) hand cleaner • Small bottle of liquid hand soap (antibacterial or antimicrobial type) • Street map • Stethoscope • Blood pressure cuff • Thermometer, thermometer sheaths • Pen light • Tongue depressors, applicators, band aids, adhesive tape, cotton balls, paper tape, 2 × 2 and 4 × 4 dressings if you are responsible for simple dressings • Alcohol and povidone-iodine swabs • Safety pins • Newspapers • Disposable, plastic aprons	• Paper bag • Plastic trash bags (medium and/or large) • Small plastic bags • Lubricant jelly or vaseline • Bandage scissors • Rubber bands • Gloves • Resuscitation mask • N95 mask • Goggles or face shield • Finger and toenail clippers in sheath • Orange sticks • Emery boards • Household disinfectant • Perineal cleanser ("peri-wash") • Baby wipes • Paper towels (carry a few folded dispenser towels, not an entire roll) • Personal care items as needed for ADL care

TIME MANAGEMENT

There are several actions you can take to make the best use of your time:

- Be sure you have everything you need for your assignments before you leave home.
- Have a work plan in mind before you arrive at the client's home.
- Organize your supplies before you begin your assignment.
- Avoid being distracted by the family.
- Call your next client if you find you will be arriving later than expected.
- Avoid getting bogged down in tasks that you are not expected to perform.

PERSONAL SAFETY

Personal safety is always a concern for home care workers. Thousands of nursing personnel make daily home care visits, and incidents of violence are few. However, you must trust your own instincts. If something does not feel right, it probably isn't. Other ways of protecting your own safety are:

- Be alert to conditions and people around you.
- Inform your employer promptly if you believe unsafe conditions exist.
- Map out the route in advance.
- Inform the client what time you will be arriving.
- Lock your purse in the trunk of your car at the beginning of your day.
- Use a "fanny pack" for essentials such as driver's license and pens.
- Wear scrubs or clothing that identifies you as a nursing caregiver.
- Wear your name badge.
- In potentially dangerous areas, find out if you can make joint visits with a coworker or use an escort.

- If neighbors, relatives, or others become a safety problem, make visits when they are away from the home.
- If a client suggests a family member escort you, accept the offer, but never get into someone else's car.
- Keep your gas tank full.
- Avoid parking on deserted streets or in dark areas.
- Keep your car windows up and doors locked at all times.
- Attend classes on personal safety and self-defense.
- Consider purchasing a cell phone.

SAFETY IN THE HOME

Your first visit to the home gives you an opportunity to check for safety factors. Tell a family member or supervising nurse about safety problems. Things to call to the attention of the supervising nurse include:

- Furniture or other items that obstruct a client's walkway
- Electrical cords that could cause the client to fall
- Stair railings and stair treads that need repair
- Unstable or lightweight chairs
- Highly polished floors that may be slippery
- The need to lock up specific items if the client is disoriented
- Loose scatter rugs, which might cause a fall as the client ambulates
- Lack of smoke detectors and a fire extinguisher
- Overloaded electrical outlets
- Ambulatory aids that need repair or replacement
- Family or client smoking when oxygen is being used in the home

Keep a list of emergency numbers close to the telephone.

ASSISTING WITH MEDICATIONS

Guidelines for Supervising Self-Administration of Medications

- The medicine must be taken at the correct time. Note whether it should be taken before meals, with food, or after meals.
- Check the expiration date to be sure the medicine is not outdated.
- Note whether the client is also taking over-the-counter medications (nonprescription) and check with the nurse to find out whether these medications will interact with the prescription drugs.
- Perform any monitoring activities required, such as checking the pulse, the blood pressure, or the blood sugar, *before* the drug is taken.
- Note how much medication is left in the container. Follow your instructions for getting the prescription refilled so that the patient does not run out.

INFECTION CONTROL

- Use good hand-washing technique.
- Apply the principles of standard precautions.
- Wear latex gloves for patient care if contact with blood, body fluids, mucous membranes, or nonintact skin is likely.
- Wear utility gloves when cleaning environmental surfaces or doing laundry contaminated with blood, body fluids, secretions, or excretions.

SUBACUTE CARE

TAKING VITAL SIGNS IN THE SUBACUTE UNIT

Patients in the subacute unit require close monitoring of their vital signs. When taking patients' vital signs, remember the following:

- Avoid taking blood pressure on the side affected by a stroke.
- Avoid taking blood pressure in an arm with a dialysis graft or shunt.
- Avoid taking blood pressure in an arm with an IV.
- Avoid taking blood pressure on the side where a patient has recently had a breast removed.
- Avoid taking an oral temperature on patients with tubes in their nose or mouth.
- Report abnormal vital signs to the nurse immediately.
- If patients are connected to electronic devices for vital sign monitoring, respond to alarms immediately.

CARING FOR PATIENTS CONNECTED TO SPECIAL EQUIPMENT

- Do not disconnect a device without specific instructions.
- Avoid accidentally moving, bumping, or disconnecting the equipment.
- Avoid bending, kinking, or placing traction on tubes entering surgical incisions or body cavities.
- In most cases, you will not be permitted to adjust or regulate the equipment.

- If an alarm sounds on a piece of equipment, respond immediately. Notify the nurse without delay.

CENTRAL VENOUS LINE

IV therapy can also be administered through a central venous (CV) catheter. A special catheter is inserted into a vein near the patient's collar bone (see Figure 39-1).

Total Parenteral Nutrition

Total parenteral nutrition (TPN) is also called hyperalimentation. TPN is given to a patient whose bowel needs complete rest. Patients receiving TPN may need to be weighed daily or every other day. This should be done at the same time of day, with the patient wearing the same type of clothing.

The catheter tip ends in or near the heart chamber.

- Be sure the tubing is not obstructed or kinked.
- Be very careful to avoid dislodging the tubing when moving or caring for the patient.
- If the line breaks or is accidentally pulled loose, clamp the tube next to the patient's body.
- Keep the clamp readily available and visible at all times.

When caring for patients with a central venous catheter, notify the nurse immediately if:

- You see blood in the IV tubing

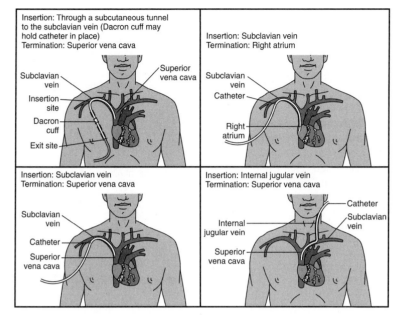

Insertion: Through a subcutaneous tunnel to the subclavian vein (Dacron cuff may hold catheter in place)
Termination: Superior vena cava

Subclavian vein
Superior vena cava
Insertion site
Dacron cuff
Exit site

Insertion: Subclavian vein
Termination: Right atrium

Subclavian vein
Catheter
Right atrium

Insertion: Subclavian vein
Termination: Superior vena cava

Subclavian vein
Catheter
Superior vena cava

Insertion: Internal jugular vein
Termination: Superior vena cava

Catheter
Subclavian vein
Internal jugular vein
Superior vena cava

Figure 39-1 Locations for insertion of central venous catheters.

- The patient has an elevated temperature or experiences chills
- You observe swelling or redness around the collarbone or near the infusion site
- The patient complains of pain in the neck or chest
- The patient becomes short of breath or develops elevated blood pressure or edema
- The catheter is broken or cracked
- The alarm sounds on the IV infusion pump

PAIN MANAGEMENT PROCEDURES

Patient-Controlled Analgesia

Patient-controlled analgesia (PCA) is used for acute, chronic, or postoperative pain. Analgesia means pain relief. The patient pushes the PCA buttons at times of discomfort. The pump has preset controls to prevent accidental medication overdose.

Report to the nurse if you note any change in the patient's:
- Level of consciousness
- Rate and pattern of respirations
- Pupil size
- Skin color

Other complications of this therapy that you should report to the nurse are:
- Nausea and/or vomiting
- Inability to urinate or difficulty urinating
- Excessive drowsiness
- Confusion
- Itching
- Preset pump alarm sounds

Constipation is a common side effect of narcotic medications. Problems can become serious if not carefully monitored. Encourage patients to eat fiber foods on trays, drink liquids, and be as active as possible in keeping with the plan of care. Carefully monitor and document the patient's bowel activity. Report patient complaints or signs of constipation to the nurse.

Pain Management with an Epidural Catheter

Patients receiving continuous epidural analgesia receive stable, consistent doses of pain medication rather than experiencing the peaks and valleys associated with most other control methods.

The patient may have leg numbness and weakness for the first 24 hours after the catheter is inserted. Limited mobility in areas not affected by the medication and decreased blood pressure when rising from bed are also common reactions.

Nursing Assistant Actions

- Instruct the patient to call for assistance in getting out of bed.
- Elevate the head of the bed 30 or 40 degrees.
- Monitor the patient's vital signs frequently.

Report to the nurse at once if:

- The catheter becomes dislodged from the insertion site.
- You note changes in respiration rate and pattern.
- The patient complains of itching.
- The patient vomits or complains of nausea.
- Dressings covering the catheter become wet from leaking or an external cause.
- Respirations decrease to 12 or below.
- Oxygen saturation drops below 90%.
- There is a decreased level of consciousness.

- The patient develops urinary retention; patient complains of need to urinate but cannot.
- The patient has low blood pressure (hypotension).
- The patient has hives.
- The patient has a rapid pulse (tachycardia).
- Redness, warmth, tenderness, swelling, itching, or drainage occurs at the catheter insertion site.
- The patient complains of inability to move legs.
- The patient complains of severe low back pain.
- The patient complains of a change in sensation or motor function.

Implantable Medication Pumps

Implantable medication pumps are sometimes used for long-term medication delivery in adults and children. The pumps are surgically placed under the abdominal skin, and medications are infused directly into the cerebrospinal fluid.

The patient may remain on bedrest for 2 to 20 hours after surgery, depending on physician preference and patient response.

Nursing Assistant Actions

- The nurse may instruct you to apply a cool application or ice pack to the site where the catheter tunnels under the skin.
- If you are assisting the patient with transfers, avoid using the transfer belt until the surgical site is well healed (usually several months after surgery, according to physician order and facility policy).

Notify the nurse if the patient:

- Has decreased responsiveness
- Has respirations of 12 or below
- Has a temperature over 100°F orally

- Complains of headache
- Experiences fluid leakage
- Develops a collection of blood or fluid under the skin at the insertion site
- Has redness, warmth, tenderness, swelling, itching, or drainage at the surgical site
- Complains of a feeling of tightness over the pump site
- Is unable to move the legs
- Has sudden loss of bowel or bladder control

CARING FOR SUBACUTE PATIENTS WITH RESPIRATORY CONDITIONS

Signs and symptoms to report to the nurse that may indicate problems with oxygen use are:
- Unusual skin color, such as dusky, pale, blue, or gray
- Unusual color of the lips, mucous membranes, nail beds, or lining or roof of the mouth
- Cool, clammy skin
- Slow, rapid, or irregular breathing
- Shortness of breath or difficulty breathing
- Noisy breathing
- Gasping for breath
- Wet respirations, rattling in the lungs
- Choking on secretions
- Changes in mental status, including decreased responsiveness, drowsiness, sleepiness for no apparent reason, restlessness, increased confusion
- Tachycardia

Capillary Refill

Capillary refill is an indication of the patient's peripheral circulation and shows how well the tissues are being nourished with oxygen. Delayed capillary refill indicates a problem with oxygen delivery. Perform a capillary refill check on all four extremities, or according to facility policy. Skin color should return to normal within 2 to 3 seconds in all patients. The color should be restored to the nail bed in the length of time it takes to say the words "capillary refill." If it takes longer than 3 seconds, inform the nurse.

The Pulse Oximeter

The pulse oximeter is an instrument that measures the level of saturation of the patient's hemoglobin with oxygen.
- Before applying the pulse oximeter, check the patient's oxygen, if being used.
- Document the liter flow.
- The pulse oximeter is attached to the patient's skin with a sensor. The finger and toe sensors work best with dark-skinned patients.
- The physician will order what he or she wants the minimum oxygen saturation to be. The nurse will give you this information.
- *A measurement of 95% to 100% is considered normal.*
- *Readings below 90% suggest complications.*
- *When the reading reaches 85%, there may not be enough oxygen for the tissues.*
- *Readings below 70% are life-threatening.*

Monitoring the Patient

If the patient's vital signs or appearance change significantly from your baseline values, notify the nurse promptly. Also inform the nurse immediately if the patient's pulse oximetry value is less than the level ordered by the physician. Monitor the patient's oxygen, if used, each time you are in the room. Make sure it is set at the liter flow ordered by the physician. Rotate the position of the finger sensor at least every 4 hours. A spring-clip sensor should be moved every 2 hours. Rotating the location of the sensor reduces the risk of skin breakdown and complications related to pressure.

Oxygen Therapy

Oxygen is a prescription item, and a physician order is necessary to administer it to a patient. The physician will order additional oxygen to be given through an oxygen delivery system. He or she will specify how much oxygen to use and the method of delivery. Depending on your facility policy, oxygen may also be given at the nurse's discretion, according to protocol or clinical practice guidelines. You should not start, stop, or change the flow rate of oxygen. Refer to Chapter 9 of your book for guidelines on caring for patients receiving oxygen therapy.

CARING FOR THE PATIENT RECEIVING DIALYSIS TREATMENTS

Dialysis is a process by which the blood is artificially cleansed of liquid wastes when the kidneys are unable to remove the wastes.

Hemodialysis

You need to be aware that the patient on dialysis will:
- Have fluid restrictions.
- Have dietary restrictions for calories, sodium, protein, potassium, calcium, and phosphorus.
- Need all fluid intake and output measured accurately and recorded.
- Need to be weighed regularly at the same time of day and with the same type of clothing.
- Need to be monitored and have vital signs taken frequently after

dialysis. Avoid taking blood pressure in the arm used for dialysis.
- Possibly be weak when they return from dialysis. Monitor them closely when they ambulate. Watch for dizziness and loss of balance.

Report to the nurse if the patient has:
- Swelling (edema) of the hands, feet, or face
- Changes in vital signs
- Changes in weight
- A change in intake or output measurements
- Shortness of breath
- Complaints of pain at the site of the fistula or graft
- Dizziness
- Hypotension

Peritoneal Dialysis

Notify the nurse if there are any changes in vital signs. Other signs and symptoms to report to the nurse are:
- The dialysate that returns appears bloody or has blood clots in the solution.
- The patient complains of abdominal pain.
- The dressing becomes wet or soiled.
- Fluid leaks around the insertion site.
- The tubing or catheter is disconnected.
- The solution does not appear to be running or is running very slowly.
- The drainage container is almost full.
- The patient is weak or unsteady.
- The patient has low blood pressure or complains of dizziness.
- The patient is short of breath or complains of difficulty breathing.

ONCOLOGY TREATMENTS

Oncology is the care and treatment of persons with cancer. Cancer may be treated with surgery, radiation, chemotherapy, or a combination of any of these.

Radiation Therapy

When caring for patients receiving radiation therapy:

• Report signs of redness, pain, or peeling of the skin in the area being treated.

• Do not remove markings made on the skin for treatment purposes.

• Do not use any heat or cold treatments on the area being treated.

• Wash the area only with tepid water and a soft washcloth; do not apply any soaps, powders, deodorants, perfumes, makeup, lotions, or skin preparations to the area.

• Instruct the patient to avoid wearing tight clothing over the area.

Chemotherapy

Chemotherapy is the use of drugs to kill cancer cells within the body. The person receiving chemotherapy may have side effects such as nausea, vomiting, anorexia (loss of appetite), or alopecia (loss of hair). Respect the patient's wishes regarding personal appearance. Assist with modesty, head coverings, caps, or scarves as the patient desires. Patients receiving chemotherapy may fear the outcome of their disease and need a great deal of emotional support. Be a good listener.

WOUND MANAGEMENT

Some patients require wound management for severe pressure ulcers, burns, or surgical wounds. Notify the nurse if any of the following occur:

• The wound appears red or swollen or has increased drainage.

• The dressing becomes saturated with drainage from the wound.

• The wound drainage has a foul odor.

• The patient complains of increased pain in the wound.

• The wound dressing becomes wet or soiled or falls off.

• The wound dressing accidentally becomes contaminated with urine or stool.

DOCUMENTATION OF CARE IN THE SUBACUTE UNIT

The main purpose of documentation is to provide a record of the patient's care. Documentation must reflect the patient's progress toward stated care plan goals and response to treatment provided. You will be responsible for documenting the services you provide. You may also be required to document the patient's response to these services. If you are working with patients on special restorative nursing or therapy programs, you may be required to document additional information. Avoid subjective terms, such as "good," "fair," or "poor." Generally, documentation about the patient's response to services or progress toward care plan goals must be stated in measurable terms, such as:

• "Ambulated 50 feet in hallway with walker."

• "Ate 90% of breakfast meal."

• "Consumed 1,775 ml of fluid orally this shift."

REHABILITATION AND RESTORATIVE SERVICES

The goals of rehabilitation and restorative care are to:

- Increase the patient's physical abilities to his or her optimum level of function. This may include mobility skills and the ability to carry out activities of daily living (ADLs).
- Prevent complications such as pressure sores and contractures.
- Maintain the patient's current abilities.
- Help the patient adapt to limitations imposed by a disability.
- Increase the patient's quality of life.

THE ROLE OF THE NURSING ASSISTANT IN REHABILITATION

The nursing assistant who works in rehabilitation will assist the nurses with:

- Procedures to prevent complications
- Mobility skills
- Bathing and personal care procedures
- Bowel and bladder training programs
- Maintaining the patient's nutritional status
- Programs to increase the patient's independence

PRINCIPLES OF REHABILITATION

Four principles form the foundation for successful rehabilitation or restorative care.

- *Treatment begins as soon as possible.*
- *Stress the patient's ability, not disability.*
- *Activity strengthens, and inactivity weakens.*
- *Treat the whole person.*

The elements of successful rehabilitation and restorative care require that members of the team:

- Have a positive attitude about the patients and their abilities
- Have confidence in their own abilities as caregivers
- Be willing to learn from other care providers, patients, and their families
- Use problem-solving skills in place of unproductive coping methods
- Use all available tools and resources to give effective care
- Work with other staff as team members
- Realize that ideal working conditions seldom exist, but strive to bring ideal and real close together
- Continually learn and acquire new skills by participating in educational programs
- Accept the need for change to improve the quality of care for all patients

COMPLICATIONS FROM INACTIVITY

People with disabilities may be unable to move about at will. The inactivity or immobility can result in

numerous complications affecting body systems:
1. Musculoskeletal System
   - Muscles become weak and atrophy (decrease in size and strength).
   - Contractures form.
   - Disuse osteoporosis develops.
2. Integumentary System
   - Pressure areas develop over bony prominences.
3. Cardiovascular System
   - The heart takes longer to return to a normal pace after activity.
   - Blood does not circulate as efficiently as usual.
   - Thrombus (blood clot) and embolus may develop.
   - Edema may be caused by lack of movement.
   - The heart may work harder to pump blood through the body.
   - Changes in the blood vessels may cause dizziness and fainting when the patient is placed in the upright position.
4. Respiratory System
   - The lungs do not expand fully.
   - Secretions collect in the lungs and cause pneumonia.
   - Respiratory tract infections are more common.
5. Gastrointestinal System
   - Appetite decreases, causing weight loss.
   - The risk of pressure sores increases with weight loss and lack of nutrition.
   - Peristalsis slows down, causing indigestion and constipation.
   - Indigestion and heartburn may result if the patient is not positioned properly for meals.
   - The patient is at risk for choking unless positioned upright during and after meals.

6. Urinary System
   - The bladder does not empty completely, increasing the risk of bladder infection.
   - Incontinence may occur.
   - Urinary stones can develop from calcium in the bloodstream resulting from osteoporosis.
7. Nervous System
   - Weakness and limited mobility may occur.
   - Insomnia may result from sleeping too much during the day.
8. Psychosocial Reaction
   - Depression.
   - Disorientation.
   - Irritability, boredom, and lethargy.

RESTORATIVE PROGRAMS

If the patient has the potential to relearn an ADL and is motivated to try, a restorative program is planned.

Approaches Used in Restorative Programs

Which approach to use should be indicated on the care plan. It is important that the same approach be used consistently.

- *Setup.* Patients with self-care deficits are not able to set up or prepare for activities of daily living. You may need to provide the setup.
- *Verbal cues.* The care provider uses short, simple phrases to prompt the patient. If a complete task, such as washing the entire face, is overwhelming, break it down into a series of smaller tasks, such as washing the forehead, then the left cheek, and so forth.
- *Hand-over-hand technique.* Place your hand over the patient's hand and guide him or her through the activity.

• *Demonstration.* Act out what you want the patient to do.

Adaptive devices are sometimes used to simplify an ADL. Adaptive devices are ordinary items that have been modified for use by patients with various types of problems. Not all patients are candidates for restorative programs. For those who are not, the goals are to prevent complications and maintain remaining abilities as long as possible. Some patients reach the point where even maintenance is difficult. We are then basically concerned with preventing complications.

The Restorative Environment

All patients benefit from living in an environment that attempts to improve the quality of life. The interdisciplinary team can help promote this environment:

• Give the patient a sense of control and opportunities to make decisions.

• Remember that mental and physical activity are essential to the patient's well-being.

• Encourage and assist patients to be well dressed and well groomed.

• Use touch freely in appropriate ways with patients.

• Provide cues for orientation throughout the building.

• Respect the patient's identity, individuality, and privacy at all times.

• Respect and understand the patient's sexuality and need for intimacy.

• Give patients opportunities to help others.

• Encourage and assist patients to remain a part of the community.

• Create an environment that is safe, serene, and colorful.

Guidelines for Implementing Restorative Programs

• Know why the patient has the self-care deficit.

• Keep your directions simple but not childish.

• Avoid distractions. Do the ADL in a private area.

• Use adaptive devices consistently and correctly.

• Do not show impatience. Be encouraging and give praise.

• Treat the patient with dignity at all times.

• Realize that the patient's progress may be uneven and inconsistent.

• Avoid statements such as, "You *can't* use your right hand." Instead say, "You *can* use your left hand."

• Allow the patient to struggle a little, but avoid letting it progress to the point of frustration before you step in to assist.

• Do the task at the time of day it is normally done. For example, most men shave in the morning.

• Make the task part of the regular routine so it is purposeful. Avoid making it look like "busy work."

• Use the care plan approaches each time the task must be done. Some things are done several times each day.

• Compliment the patient for making progress even if his or her gains are small.

THE OBSTETRICAL PATIENT AND NEONATE

STAGES OF PREGNANCY

There are three stages of pregnancy:
- Prenatal (before birth)
- Labor and delivery
- Postpartum (after birth)

The nursing assistant, who is specially trained, helps provide care and support throughout each phase.

PRENATAL CARE

The care of the mother begins in the prenatal period, when she first learns she is pregnant. You may meet her as you work in a doctor's office or in an obstetrical (pregnancy) clinic.

A normal pregnancy lasts about 280 days and is divided into trimesters (3 months). Each trimester is noted by specific signs and symptoms. The care of the mother throughout pregnancy is important to ensure the birth of a healthy baby. The first trimester is an especially critical time. During the first 3 months, the fetus is very susceptible to the negative effects of tobacco, alcohol, caffeine, and other drugs, as well as to viruses and bacteria. Exposure to any of these may cause physical and/or mental harm to the developing fetus. The pregnant woman is usually advised to visit the physician, nurse practitioner, or midwife at least once a month during the first trimester. During the first visit, the examiner will complete a very thorough history and physical examination.

Visits become more frequent as the pregnancy progresses. Routine procedures during the visits include:
- Weighing the mother
- Taking the blood pressure and pulse
- Urine testing
- Counseling and teaching the mother about diet, lifestyle, and signs and symptoms that she should report to the physician
- Palpating the abdomen to check fetal size
- Listening for fetal heart tones

You should call anything unusual to the attention of the nurse. Examples of items to report are:
- Complaints of persistent headache
- Elevated blood pressure
- Vaginal bleeding
- Complaints of dizziness
- Swelling of the hands and feet

LABOR AND DELIVERY

At the end of 40 weeks (within 2 weeks more or less), the signs of impending labor will be noted:
- Engagement or lightening occurs (the fetus moves downward—sometimes known as "dropping").
- Mucus plug is expelled from the cervix.
- Dilation of cervix begins.
- Amniotic membranes may rupture just before actual labor begins or may rupture during labor.
- Uterine contractions begin
  - Irregular at first

– Stronger, more regular, and closer together as labor progresses

The mother is told during her pregnancy when she should go to hospital.

Dilation

The dilation (opening) stage begins with the first regular uterine contractions. It ends when the cervix is fully dilated or opened. This may take 18 to 24 hours in a first pregnancy. As the labor progresses, the cervix also thins (effaces) so that the fetus may move downward into the birth canal and out of the mother's body. The degree of dilation at any given time is measured by the nurse or physician, who places a gloved finger in the patient's vagina and measures (approximately) the size of the cervical opening and amount of effacement. This procedure is called vaginal examination.

Expulsion

Expulsion stage is the period extending from the point of full cervical dilation until the baby is delivered. This may be 1 to 2 hours or more.

The baby moves down the birth canal. The mother is encouraged to help the process by "bearing down" with her abdominal muscles with each contraction. During delivery, it may be necessary to enlarge the vaginal opening. This is done by making a cut—called an episiotomy—in the perineum. The episiotomy is sutured (sewn up) after the delivery.

Forceps may be used at this stage to assist in delivery of the head. Once delivered, the baby is held head down to clear the respiratory tract. The baby is then usually placed on the mother's abdomen while the cord is clamped and cut. In addition:

- An Apgar score is determined. This score is used to evaluate a newborn at 1 minute, 5 minutes, and 10 minutes after delivery on five qualities. The higher the score, the better the baby's condition.
- The mother is encouraged to hold her newborn, now called a neonate, to establish emotional bonding. This is done even when the baby is delivered by cesarean section.

Placental Stage

The placental stage lasts from delivery of the baby through the delivery of the placenta. This is a short period. The placenta is usually delivered within an hour of the delivery of the baby.

In this stage, the placenta separates from the wall of the uterus. Uterine contractions push it downward and out through the birth canal. After delivery of the placenta:

- If an episiotomy was needed, it is repaired.
- The mother's uterus is checked for firmness. Drugs may be given to help it contract to control bleeding.
- Both mother and child are identified with numbered identification bands before being separated.
- The baby is footprinted along with the mother's thumbprint.
- The baby's eyes are treated to prevent infection.

Cesarean Birth

Cesarean section is another way of delivering a baby. The baby is delivered through an incision in the abdomen rather than through the birth canal. Between 20% and 30% of all births in the United States occur this way.

A spinal anesthetic or epidural is administered before the surgery. This type of procedure introduces the drugs into the cerebrospinal fluid and blocks sensation from the upper abdomen down to the toes. Until the anesthetic wears off, the patient will not be able to either feel or move her legs.

POSTPARTUM CARE

You may be assigned to assist in caring for the mother during the postpartum period.

* With other team members, you will assist the mother from the stretcher into bed.
* A protective pad (Chux) may be placed under the patient's buttocks.
* Always wear gloves and follow standard precautions when caring for the postpartum patient. There is a high probability of contact with blood, mucous membranes, urine, stool, and breast milk. All of these body fluids are considered potentially infectious.

Anesthesia

If an anesthetic was used, follow the procedures for postoperative care of surgical patients.

* Keep the patient flat on her back.
* Make sure the patient has a fresh gown and clean bed linen.
* Check blood pressure, pulse, and respirations as ordered until the patient is stable.
* Continue to monitor vital signs every 4 hours for 24 hours.
* If the patient complains of being cold, an extra blanket may provide comfort. If the patient does not become comfortable, inform the nurse.
* Record the first voiding. Inform the nurse if the patient has not voided by the end of your shift.

Drainage

Carefully check the condition of the perineum and the perineal pad for the amount and color of drainage. Always wear gloves during this procedure.

* When removing the pad, always lift it away from the body from front to back.
* Red vaginal discharge, called lochia, is expected. Lochia rubra is the name given to discharge the first 3 days after delivery.

Initially, the lochia is bright red and moderate in amount. Over the next week, the lochia will decrease and become pink to pink-brown in color. A discharge that is yellowish white or brown may continue for 1 to 3 weeks after delivery and then stop.

Note and report:

* Signs of tenderness
* Signs of inflammation
* Presence of an episiotomy
* Presence of large blood clots
* Foul-smelling lochia
* Saturation of a pad in 15 to 30 minutes

The Uterus

The size and firmness of the uterus should be checked and reported. A soft and enlarging uterus indicates excessive bleeding.

Massaging

The top of the uterus, the fundus, is massaged in a circular fashion while the opposite hand is held against the pubic bone. Massaging the fundus stimulates the uterine muscles to contract, firming the uterus.

Measuring Height of Uterus

The level of the fundus is measured by placing the fingers lengthwise across the abdomen between the fundus and the navel. On the first postpartal day, the level of the fundus is usually at the umbilicus or one to two fingers' width below.

Cramping

As the uterus begins to return to its normal size (involution), the patient may experience strong uterine contractions or cramps. Cramping may also be associated with breastfeeding. This is normal, but be sure to report any complaints of pain to the nurse, who can administer medication for relief.

Voiding

The new mother should be encouraged to void within the first 4 to 8 hours after the delivery. Check carefully for signs of urine retention. These include:

- A uterus that is unusually high or pushed to one side
- Swelling just above the pubis
- Complaints of urgency (the need to void), but with voidings of 200 ml or less

Be sure to report:

- Signs of possible urine retention immediately, so the patient's recovery will not be impeded
- Any inability to void within the first 8 hours postpartum
- Voidings of less than 100 ml

TOILETING AND PERINEAL CARE

The mother may be:

- Provided with a squeezable bottle filled with warm tap water.
- Instructed to rinse the genitals and perineum after voiding or defecating.
- Instructed to gently pat, not wipe, the perineal area containing the stitches with tissue or special medicated pads—once only, from front to back. The tissue is discarded in the toilet.
- Taught to wash her hands before applying a fresh perineal pad.

- Taught not to touch the inside of the perineal pad.
- Infection occurs in about 6% of all postpartum patients. When assisting patients with toileting, teach the patient to stand up before flushing the toilet to prevent spraying with contaminated water. Inform the nurse promptly if a patient has an elevated temperature, chills, foul-smelling lochia, or other signs and symptoms of infection.

If the perineum is very uncomfortable:

- Specially medicated pads may be used for cleansing. The procedure is always the same—front to back and discard.
- Anesthetic sprays may be ordered.
- Ice packs may be used to reduce edema and give comfort.

Patients should be cautioned to apply anesthetics and ointments after cleansing. Sitting may be uncomfortable when an episiotomy has been performed. Instruct the mother to squeeze her buttocks together and hold them in this position until she is seated upright. This reduces tension on the suture line.

Breast Care

The mother's first milk is called colostrum. The colostrum:

- Is watery.
- Carries protective antibodies to the child.
- Usually begins to flow about 12 hours after delivery. Lactation, the flow of milk, does not begin until the second or third postpartum day.

Keeping the breasts clean is especially important when the mother is planning to breast-feed her baby.

- The mother's hands and nipples should be washed just prior to feeding the baby.

- During the shower, the mother should wash her breasts, using a circular motion from the nipples outward.
- Creams are sometimes used between feedings to help the nipples remain supple.
- Breast pads absorb milk leakage. They should be changed frequently.
- The breasts should be supported by a well-fitted brassiere.

Even if a mother chooses not to breast-feed, the breasts should be washed daily with soap and water.

NEONATAL CARE

After the newborn is admitted to the nursery, some procedures not carried out in the delivery room are completed. The physician or nurse will examine the baby and make an evaluation of the baby's condition, or status.

In the nursery the baby's vital signs are determined. Measurements of length and weight are also taken.

When the newborn's status becomes stable:

- If the eyes were not treated with silver nitrate drops or antibiotics in the delivery room, or the footprints were not taken, these procedures are done at this time.
- The baby is cleaned. Sometimes an admission bath using an antiseptic soap or oil is administered, but procedures for bathing newborns vary from hospital to hospital. In some hospitals, the bath is omitted, and the cheesy material known as *vernix caseosa* is allowed to remain on the skin. The area around the umbilical cord is carefully cleaned with a solution prescribed by the facility.
- The baby must be kept warm because a newborn's temperature has not yet stabilized. The baby is dressed according to facility policy.

A stockinette cap is placed on the head because much body heat can be lost through this surface.

- The baby is placed in a crib or isolette.
- Feeding is not usually started for 4 to 6 hours after birth. During these hours, the baby is monitored and observed carefully for successful, independent life. After 12 hours, the baby is either taken to the mother's breast or started on feedings of glucose and water. Babies whose mothers are unable to feed will be fed in the nursery.
- Male babies may be circumcised before discharge. In circumcision, the excess tissue (foreskin) is cut from the tip of the penis. This procedure is usually performed based on the parents' personal choices, as well as cultural, ethnic, and religious traditions.
- Babies who are jaundiced may have their eyes protected and be placed under a special light (bili light) to help clear the levels of bilirubin in the skin.

Post Circumcision Care

- The circumcision should be checked each time the diaper is changed and should be a routine part of that care.
- Observe the incision site for bleeding and report anything unusual.
- The crib identification should note the new circumcision.
- A note should also be included on the nursery record regarding the condition of the circumcision and first voiding after circumcision.

Handling the Infant

Take care when lifting, carrying, and positioning an infant. Remember to:

- Lift the baby by grasping the legs securely with one hand while slipping the other hand under the baby's back to support the head and neck.

• Hold the baby securely.

• Support the head, neck, and back at all times.

• Back through doorways when carrying a baby.

• Never turn your back on an infant who is on an unprotected surface.

Infant Security

All infants must be identified to prevent inadvertent switching, misidentification, and abduction. The infant, mother, and sometimes the father are given matching wrists band. Be sure to check the identification bands each time you bring the infant to the room. Crib cards are also used for infant identification. Follow your facility policies for checking identification.

Sadly, a number of infant abductions occur each year. As part of the security measures in place to help prevent abduction, nursing personnel are expected to wear a photo identification badge. Reinforce your identity and position to the mothers each time you provide care. The mother is instructed not to hand the infant over to someone she does not know. If the infant must be transported to another area of the hospital, nursing staff must remain with the child, then return him or her to the nursery. Adhere to your facility policies for preventing infant abduction.

DISCHARGE

To carry out the discharge procedure from the facility:

• Match the baby's identification with the mother's.

• Dress the child in his or her own clothing.

• Wrap the baby in a blanket, using the technique of "papoosing."

• Check to be sure that the mother has received and understands any special discharge instructions. If not, inform the nurse.

• Check to be sure equipment or needed formula is ready when the parents and newborn are ready to go home.

• Transport the mother, carrying her baby, by wheelchair to the discharge area.

• Make sure the infant is strapped into a properly secured car seat. Stay with the family until they leave.

• Record discharge information on the charts of both mother and child. Include the condition of each and the time of release.

THE PEDIATRIC PATIENT

CARING FOR INFANTS (BIRTH TO AGE 1)

- The infant communicates with his or her cry and body movements.
- The cry can vary depending on needs.
- The caregiver will learn to interpret the meanings of the cry by caring for the infant.
- Infants respond to voices, faces, and touch.
- Talk to the infant whenever you are giving personal care such as bathing, feeding, or holding.

Refer to Table 42-1 for developmental milestones.

The Waking Hours

- Provide age-appropriate toys, such as colorful mobiles, rattles, and mirrors.

Routine Procedures

- Organize care so the infant can digest his or her food, then sleep after eating.
- Avoid moving the infant unnecessarily, as this may cause vomiting.
- In organizing the care, you would weigh, bathe, diaper, and then dress the infant. Then change the crib linens and feed the infant.

Feeding

Sucking provides the infant with a pleasant sensation, whether or not it provides food. The amount of time needed for sucking will vary with each infant. Always provide the infant with the opportunity to suck. This is even more important if the infant cannot eat.

When feeding an infant:

- Hold the infant unless there is a medical reason not to.
- If an infant cannot be held, you should still hold the bottle for him or her during feeding.
- An infant should never be left in a crib with a bottle propped in his or her mouth.
- Holding the infant during feeding also allows close physical contact with the person providing the feeding.
- The infant should be burped during and after feeding.

Note: *If an infant cannot be fed, he or she should still be held and allowed to suck on a pacifier unless a medical reason prevents removal of the infant from the crib.*

Breast-Feeding

If the rooming-in or visiting mother is breast-feeding, she should be directed to an area where she can be assured of privacy as well as comfort. As a nursing assistant, you may be responsible for weighing the infant before and after feeding, according to your hospital policy.

Table 42-1	NORMAL AGE FOR ATTAINMENT OF MAJOR DEVELOPMENTAL MILESTONES		
AGE	MOTOR SKILL	LANGUAGE	ADAPTIVE BEHAVIOR
4-6 wks.	Head lifted from prone position and turned from side to side	Cries	Smiles
4 mo.	No head lag when pulled to sitting from supine position Tries to grasp large objects	Sounds of pleasure	Smiles, laughs aloud, and shows pleasure re familiar objects or persons
5 mo.	Voluntary grasp with both hands	Primitive sounds: "ah goo"	Smiles at self in mirror
6 mo.	Grasps with one hand Rolls prone to supine Sits with support	Range of sounds greater	Expresses displeasure and food preference
8 mo.	Sits without support Transfers objects from hand to hand Rolls supine to prone	Combines syllables: "baba, dada, mama"	Responds to "No"
10 mo.	Sits well Creeping Stands holding onto support Finger-thumb opposition in picking up small objects		Waves "bye-bye," plays "patty-cake" and "peek-a-boo"
12 mo.	Stands holding onto support Walks with support	Says two or three words with meaning	Understands names of objects Shows interest in pictures
15 mo.	Walks alone	Several intelligible words	Requests by pointing Imitates
18 mo.	Walks up and down stairs holding support Removes clothes	Many intelligible words	Carries out simple commands
2 yrs.	Walks up and down stairs by self Runs	Two- to three-word phrases	Organized play Points to some parts of body

Source: Mary Fran Hazinski, *Nursing Care of the Critically Ill Child* (St. Louis: C.V. Mosby Company, 1984, p. 387).

Restraints

It is generally not necessary to obtain a physician's order to restrain an infant or child. Follow your facility policies. Restraints can be used for the child's safety. They are used to protect the child from injury. They are occasionally used to protect staff from injury caused by the child. Sometimes they are used to protect the child from injury by equipment used in his or her care. Review the safety precautions and guidelines for using restraints in Chapter 21 of your book. These apply to adults and children alike. Be sure to toilet the child regularly. If he or she cannot use a call signal, visually monitor and check on the child frequently. Restraints should never be tied to a crib side or bed rail, only to the bed or crib frame.

A jacket restraint is a sleeveless cloth garment that is fitted to the child's chest and crosses in the back, out of the child's reach. It has long straps that can be tied under the mattress or through a chair, allowing the child to move extremities, sit up, lie down in bed, or turn side to side without falling. An extremity restraint may be used on the child's arms, hands, legs, or feet.

Guidelines for Ensuring a Safe Environment for Infants

- Always keep crib side rails up.
- Always keep one hand on the infant when the crib side rail is down.
- Use crib bumpers or rolled blankets to prevent injury.
- Never tie balloons or toys to cribs.
- Never use toys with small removable parts or pointed objects.
- Never prop bottles.
- Never tape pacifiers in an infant's mouth.

CARING FOR TODDLERS (1–3 YEARS)

- The years between 1 and 3 can be a difficult time for a child to be hospitalized.

When caring for the toddler, allow him or her as much independence and choice as possible (within hospital policy guidelines). Avoid situations that could create a struggle between the caregiver and the child. Expect delays when the child is feeding him- or herself or bathing. Be sure to allow the toddler time to do these activities.

The Hospital Environment

It is important to provide an environment that allows as much independence and control as possible while ensuring safety. If the child is toilet trained, it is important to know the words he or she uses for urination and bowel movements. It is important to know if the child uses a potty chair or the toilet at home. You should try to provide the same arrangement for toileting in the hospital. It is not uncommon for a hospitalized child to regress. You should not be surprised if a toddler who is toilet trained starts to have "accidents" while in the hospital. Do not scold the child if this happens. The incident should be treated in a matter-of-fact manner. In addition, a hospitalized toddler may ask for a bottle or pacifier. Even though the toddler may have been weaned from them, treat the request as normal. Do not try to reason with the child.

The Toddler's Need for Autonomy

The toddler is learning to be independent and may want to feed, dress, and wash him- or herself while in the hospital. It will be your responsibility to help the toddler with these activities. You should allow the toddler to be independent, but at the same time, you must keep him or her safe.

Emotional Reaction to Illness

You must stress that the illness is not the toddler's or anyone else's fault.

To overcome anxiety about routine procedures, allow the toddler to handle the equipment whenever possible. A few extra minutes spent familiarizing the toddler with the equipment to be used may make the difference between a frightened child and an interested one.

The toddler will have a difficult time if separated from the mother. One way to prevent this is to permit the mother to room-in. If a parent is not going to stay:

- Reassure the child that he or she will not be alone.
- Tell the child the names of the caregivers.
- Introduce other caregivers.
- Whenever possible, the toddler who does not have a parent staying with him or her should be placed in a room near the nurses' station.
- Encourage parents who cannot visit to call, or you can call the parents so the child can talk to them.

Routine Activities

Routines are important to toddlers. Ask the parents to describe the child's normal day. Try to follow the child's usual schedule as much as possible for eating, naps, toileting, and other activities. Ask the parents about the child's nickname, likes, dislikes, names of siblings and pets, and anything else the parents feel the nursing assistant should know about the child.

Toddlers love to play, but because they have short attention spans, they cannot play with one toy for a long time. Plan a variety of activities to keep the toddler amused. For example:

- Finger painting
- Moving toy cars or trucks
- Coloring
- Handling blocks
- Push-pull toys
- Reading of stories

Educational toys that teach how to dress, button, and zip can also be fun for the toddler. Stethoscopes, masks, and gloves make good hospital toys because they can allow the toddler to work out his fears. Do not leave the child alone with these items because of the risk of injury.

Toddlers will not play together, but they will play near or next to each other. Temper tantrums can be common with toddlers. If they occur, ignore the tantrum as long as the child cannot hurt him- or herself or others. If a toddler is misbehaving, set limits in a firm, consistent manner.

When working with the toddler, remember that he or she is trying to be independent. Allow the child as much choice as possible. It is best to be truthful and to give simple explanations to toddlers. If the child is having a blood test, tell him or her just before it happens. It does not do any good to prepare toddlers in advance because they do not have any concept of time. Such advance warning only increases their anxiety. The toddler has natural curiosity and loves to explore. It is important to maintain a safe environment in the hospital.

Guidelines for Ensuring a Safe Environment for Toddlers

- All poisonous liquids should be kept in a locked container or cabinet.

- All open electrical sockets should have protective covers. Never leave toddlers unattended or unsupervised.
- Never leave toddlers alone in the bathtub or bathroom.
- Keep thermometers out of toddlers' reach.
- Keep crib sides and side rails up when the toddler is in bed.
- Never allow toddlers to play with balloons unless supervised.
- Avoid toys with sharp edges, long strings, or small removable parts.
- Keep doors to stair, kitchen, treatment, and storage areas closed and locked whenever possible.
- Keep doors to linen chutes locked.

Summary of Nursing Assistant Tasks When Caring for Infants and Toddlers

- Maintain a safe environment.
- Apply standard precautions if contact with blood, body fluids, mucous membranes, or nonintact skin is likely.
- Provide information to the health team through monitoring of vital-signs (temperature, pulse, and respiration), weight, intake, and output.
- Supervise and assist with routine care such as bathing, feeding, and dressing.
- Collect and test specimens.
- Assist with treatments, examinations, and procedures.
- Provide and assist with opportunities for play.
- Provide warmth, security, and affection.
- Promote independence with toddlers by providing opportunities for choices.

CARING FOR PRESCHOOL CHILDREN (3–6 YEARS)

The preschooler needs his or her independence but still needs to be safe and secure. The caregiver must provide the correct balance of independence and control for the preschooler.

Emotional Reactions to Illness

Preschoolers normally have many fears. One fear is that their body parts will be injured or changed. Therefore, it is important to use simple, honest explanations when telling the preschooler what to expect.

Fear of the dark, of nighttime, and of being alone are other normal fears for the preschooler. You can help reduce this fear by leaving a nightlight on. Another child in the room can also ease the preschooler's fears. Be sure to leave the call bell within reach. Sitting with the preschooler until he or she falls asleep will also help. Like the toddler, the preschooler can also benefit from having his or her mother room-in because the child still fears separation.

"Magical thinking" and fantasy are still present in children in this age-group. Therefore, it is important to stress to them that it is not their fault that they are sick, and that they are not sick because they were bad. The preschooler needs to know that he or she will return home and will not be forgotten and left in the hospital. Siblings should be allowed and encouraged to visit. In addition to easing separation from the family, this can be a way of assuring the child that no one is taking her place at home.

Explaining Procedures

When telling a preschooler what to expect, simple, honest explanations work best. Choose your words carefully because the preschooler takes things literally (exactly as said).

• If surgery is being planned, show and tell the child what parts of the body will be involved in the procedure.

• Preschoolers have a limited concept of time, so when you explain when something will occur, use time references that are familiar to the child (e.g., mealtime, naptime, or the time of a favorite TV show).

• Always explain to the preschooler what you are going to do. Do not assume that he or she will remember what you said earlier. The preschooler needs to maintain some control. Therefore, allow him or her to make as many decisions as possible. Provide the opportunity to make a choice.

• Allow the preschooler to do as much of his or her own care as possible, to make the child feel independent.

Activities

Imagination and fantasy are part of the preschooler's world. Imaginary playmates are normal for the preschooler and may find their way to the hospital with the child. These playmates can vary in age and sex. They often have different or unusual-sounding names. If the child talks about his or her imaginary friend, treat it matter-of-factly and listen. However, you need to be realistic. Do not say that you see or hear the playmate. Just say that you know this playmate exists only in the child's imagination.

Play is important for the hospitalized preschooler. Play may give you clues about what the child is thinking. The preschooler has become more coordinated and can enjoy activities such as puzzles, coloring, and drawing. The

preschooler enjoys imitating roles and playing with other children. Playing house or doctor is especially fun for this age-group. Hand puppets are also a good way to talk to preschoolers because the children relate easily to the character of the puppet.

You can help the preschooler deal with a hospital stay by maintaining consistency in his or her schedule and in the limits put on his or her behavior. Positive reinforcers such as hugs or stickers should be used as rewards for appropriate behavior.

Guidelines for Ensuring a Safe Environment for Preschoolers

• Keep toys from cluttering walkways to prevent falls.
• Keep side rails on bed up at night.
• Keep beds in low position.
• Keep doors to kitchen and storage areas closed.
• Keep a nightlight on.
• Never leave the child unattended in the bathtub.
• Never allow children to run with popsicles or lollipops in their mouths.

CARING FOR SCHOOL-AGE CHILDREN (6–12 YEARS)

In general, the school-age years are a time of exceptionally good health. School-age children either have had most of the childhood illnesses or have been immunized against them. The most common problems of these times involve the gastrointestinal system (for example, stomach aches), colds, and coughs. The school-age child's reaction to hospitalization will be significantly different from that of the younger child. Hospitalization can present the school-age child with an opportunity to:

- Explore a new environment
- Meet new friends
- Learn more about her body

Psychosocial Adjustment

Separation from parents will not be as difficult for the school-age child as for the younger child. However, those just entering this period may regress to preschool level. These children will need their parents' presence.

In school, the child has begun to develop relationships with other children. In the hospital, he or she may respond more to separation from peers than from the parents. It is important to give these children opportunities to communicate with their schoolmates. When possible, friends can visit.

The older school-age child may welcome the opportunity to be away from his or her parents. In this situation, the child can test newly developed skills and increase independence. Children of this age-group also need privacy—but if the parents are there, they may not get it. Some parents may need to have their child's opposition to their staying explained in this context, because they may think the child is angry with them.

Roommate selection is especially important for this age-group. A roommate of approximately the same age will act as a diversion. Because the school-age child is seeking more independence, he or she may be reluctant to ask for help even when it is needed. His or her feelings may show themselves in different ways, such as:

- Irritability.
- Hostility toward siblings.
- Other behavior problems. It is important that you, as a caregiver, observe and note these behaviors and bring them to the attention of the nurse.

Resistance to bedtime may also become a problem during these years. In the hospital, it is important to be aware of and follow the parents' rules. Learning rules is another developmental task of the school-age years.

Adjustment to Illness

By involving school-age children in their own care, you will help them to be more cooperative patients. Procedures that we routinely do without explanation or without providing options, such as using the bedpan, can be particularly upsetting to school-age children, who are trying hard to act grown-up but are not being given the chance. It is also important for a school-age child's self-esteem that you do not scold when he or she does lose self-control. It is best just to overlook the episode.

School-age children are able to reason. They also understand the impact of their illness and the potential for disability and death. These children take an active interest in health and enjoy acquiring knowledge. You can help them gain information as well as deal with their fears by explaining all procedures in simple terms.

Pain is passively accepted by the school-age child, who is able to tell you where the pain is located and what it feels like. The child will hold rigidly still, bite his lip, or clench his fists when in pain, in an effort to keep in control and to act brave. This child does well with distraction during painful procedures. During procedures, you should stay with him whenever possible to talk him through them. This child also tries to postpone all major procedures. The caregiver needs to put limits on the number of postponements the child is allowed.

Activities

Increased physical and social activities are characteristic of this period. Hospitalization does not usually provide school-age children with adequate diversions. School-age children may also miss the activities of school, although they usually deny this.

You should allow these children time during the day for their own work, such as school work and visits with friends and other patients. Having the play therapist at the hospital provide appropriate activities will help to reduce the stress the child feels.

Caregivers should encourage school-age children to take part in their own care as part of their work. Helping to make their beds or clean their rooms will make them feel useful. They should be held responsible for tasks that are within their own capabilities.

Guidelines for Ensuring a Safe Environment for School-Age Children

- Never leave poisonous materials within reach.
- Keep side rails up when children are in bed.
- Monitor toys to ensure that they are not dangerous.

Summary of Nursing Assistant Tasks and Responsibilities When Caring for Preschool and School-Age Children

- Maintain a safe environment.
- Apply standard precautions if contact with blood, body fluids, mucous membranes, or nonintact skin is likely.
- Provide information to the health care team through monitoring of vital signs (temperature, pulse, and respiration), weight, intake, and output.

- Supervise and assist with routine care.
- Collect and test specimens.
- Assist with treatments, examinations, and procedures.
- Provide warmth, security, and affection, as appropriate. Preschool and young school-age children respond well to hugs. Some older children appreciate them as well. Ask older children and adolescents if you can hug them, such as by saying, "Do you need a hug?" or "Can I give you a hug?"
- Provide opportunities and assist with age-appropriate play and activities, such as drawing or reading.

For preschoolers:

- Encourage independence with ADLs, with supervision. Assist, if necessary.

For school age children:

- Provide explanations using proper names of body parts, drawings, and books.
- Encourage socialization with other children in the same age-group.
- Provide time for school work and tutors.

CARING FOR THE ADOLESCENT (13–18 YEARS)

Adolescence is the transitional period from childhood into adulthood. Like school-age children, adolescents are relatively healthy. The major health problems of this period are usually related to the drastic physical changes that occur during this time, to accidents, to sport injuries, or to chronic and/or permanent disabilities. The adolescent is developing an identity and becoming increasingly independent. Because of this, it is important to allow the adolescent to make as many of his or her own decisions as possible. When this is not possible, keep the adolescent involved in the decision-making process.

Adolescents often have a difficult time with authority figures. You should not get into power struggles with them. Limit the restrictions on them whenever appropriate.

Adolescents may be uncooperative. The best approach is to let them know, in a nonthreatening way, what the rules are. It is best to do this at the time of admission. Speak to adolescents as you would to adults. Be as flexible as possible. The most important people to most adolescents are their friends. A hospital stay makes it more difficult for the adolescent to see friends. It is essential that you:

- Allow the adolescent time for visits.
- Permit phone calls.
- Introduce them to other patients their age.

Recognize that adolescents may not want to visit with others if illness has changed their appearance in any way. Body image is important at this age.

Use the opportunity to teach good hygiene practices if the hospitalized adolescent does not already practice them. Ask a nurse to help you if you note that this is a problem for your patient.

Keep in mind that adolescents are very aware of the changes taking place in their bodies, whether or not they can see them. It is important to provide adolescents with privacy, and to keep them covered as much as possible during procedures and examinations.

Nutrition and Activity

Adolescents go through a growth spurt. Girls are usually 2 years ahead of boys. Adequate nutrition and rest continue to be important. In the hospital, the importance of proper eating habits should be stressed to the adolescent. You should:

- Permit the adolescent to continue to make decisions about what and when he or she will eat, unless it is medically unsafe.
- Recognize that adolescent girls are often on diets. Emotional problems related to weight are common.
- Be aware that adolescents frequently skip breakfast.

It is important to explain the routines of the unit and yet provide flexibility for the adolescent.

Guidelines for Ensuring a Safe Environment for Adolescents

- Carefully check all electrical equipment that the adolescent brings to the hospital—radios, hair dryers, and so on—to ensure that it is appropriate and safe to use. Review hospital guidelines regarding use of electrical equipment with the patient.
- Reinforce to adolescents that smoking, alcohol, and other drugs are illegal and are not permitted.
- Provide assistance with showers and bathing if the patient is incapacitated or weakened in any way. The adolescent may not ask for assistance. Keep the genital area covered with a towel during a tub bath, and use a bath blanket during a bed bath and when needed before and after a shower or tub bath to drape the child for modesty.
- Reinforce the use of shoes or slippers to prevent injuries to the feet.
- Remind adolescents to keep staff informed of their whereabouts.
- Keep beds in low position to prevent falls.

Summary of Nursing Assistant Tasks and Responsibilities When Caring for Adolescents

- Maintain a safe environment.
- Apply standard precautions if contact with blood, body fluids, mucous membranes, or nonintact skin is likely.
- Orient the adolescent to unit and hospital rules.
- Provide information to the health team through monitoring of vital signs (temperature, pulse, and respiration), weight, intake, and output.
- Provide simple explanations to the adolescent.
- Assist with body hygiene to help maintain positive self-image. Remember that children of this age are very uncomfortable when private parts of their bodies are exposed. Make an effort to protect their dignity, modesty, and privacy whenever necessary.
- Collect and test specimens.
- Assist with treatment, examinations, and procedures.
- Promote independence. Allow adolescents as much control as possible over the schedule of treatments, procedures, and so on.
- Encourage socialization with other adolescents.

CARING FOR THE PATIENT WITH CANCER

CHAPTER

43

SIGNS AND SYMPTOMS OF CANCER

Each type of cancer has its own signs and symptoms. General signs and symptoms that may indicate cancer spell the word CAUTION:

C = Change in bowel or bladder habits

A = A sore that does not heal

U = Unusual bleeding or discharge

T = Thickening or lump in the breast, testicles, or any part of the body

I = Indigestion or difficulty swallowing

O = Obvious change in a wart, mole, or skin condition

N = Nagging cough or hoarseness.

Screening

Regular screening (Table 43-1) for cancer is a key to survival because the outcome is better if the disease is detected early. Screening is based on a person's age, sex, risk factors, family history, ethnicity, and history of exposure to carcinogens in the environment.

Table 43-1 SCREENING RECOMMENDATIONS

LOCATION	SCREENING TEST	AGE	FREQUENCY OF TEST
Breast	Mammogram	35–39	Baseline examination
Breast	Mammogram	40 and over	Yearly
Prostate	Rectal exam PSA blood test	50 and over	Yearly
Testicles	Exam by doctor	15 and over	Yearly
Colon/rectum	Digital rectal exam Fecal occult blood test	40 and over	Yearly
Colon/rectum	Sigmoidoscopy	50 and over	Every 3 years
Colon/rectum	Colonoscopy	50 and over	Every 5 years
Cervix	Pap smear	18 and over or at onset of sexual activity	Yearly
Skin	Skin examination	20–39	Every 3 years
Skin	Skin examination	over 40	Yearly
Mouth	Oral examination	20–39	Every 3 years
Mouth	Oral examination	over 40	Yearly

TREATMENT

Many different treatments are used for cancer. In addition, some people use alternative and complementary therapies. The type of treatment is determined by:

- Type of cancer
- Location of cancer
- Whether the cancer is malignant or benign
- Stage (how advanced the cancer is)
- General condition of the patient

Surgery

A biopsy is a minor surgery that is sometimes done to diagnose the cancer. It involves removing a small piece of tissue from a suspicious area. The tissue is sent for laboratory examination. If the biopsy is positive for cancerous cells, a surgical procedure is done with the goal of completely removing the cancer. This may involve removing all or part of an organ, such as a lung, breast, or the uterus. Lymph nodes in the area may also be removed. The surgeon removes as much cancerous tissue as possible. If removing the entire cancerous area is not possible, a portion is left and will be treated with other methods.

Reconstructive surgery may be done for cosmetic repair of an area. Sometimes this is done early, and other times it is performed a long time after the original surgery. An example of this type of surgery is breast reconstruction.

Chemotherapy

Chemotherapy uses medications or drugs to destroy the cancer. Unfortunately, healthy cells may also be destroyed. The goals of chemotherapy vary, depending on the type of cancer, stage, and situation. Goals may include:

- Completely eliminating the cancer

- Controlling and slowing the growth of cancer to prolong the patient's life
- Reducing the size of the cancer to eliminate pain and improve quality of life

Never eat, drink, or chew gum in an area where chemotherapy is being prepared. If you accidentally contact a chemotherapy drug with your hands or mucous membranes, flush well with water and seek medical attention. These drugs and the containers they are dispensed in require special handling and disposal.

Side Effects of Chemotherapy

Chemotherapy targets rapidly regenerating cells, such as cancer cells. The drugs cannot differentiate cancer cells from normal cells, so other cells that regenerate rapidly may also be affected. Other cells in the body that are commonly affected are:

- Blood cells, such as red blood cells, white blood cells, and platelets
- Hair and nail cells
- Gastrointestinal cells

Side effects of cancer drugs can range from mild to life-threatening. Patients receiving these drugs need special monitoring. Sometimes the dose and scheduling must be changed to reduce side effects. Common side effects are:

- Alopecia, or hair loss. This commonly starts within 2 weeks after chemotherapy begins. It may take up to 5 or 6 months to regrow the hair.
- Nausea and vomiting may be present, depending on the drugs used. Sometimes they occur immediately, but they may be delayed until several days after the drug is given.
- Anorexia, or loss of appetite. This is sometimes caused because the drugs cause changes in the taste buds. In some patients, loss of appetite is due to nausea.

- Anemia, a deficiency of the red blood cells. This is caused by changes in the body due to the chemotherapy drugs. Sometimes special medications are given to reverse the anemia.
- Fatigue. Patients often become very tired. Anemia and reduced red blood cells are the most likely cause.
- Low white blood cell count, which increases the risk of infection. This usually begins within a week of starting therapy and may last a long time. Precautions are taken to prevent exposure to infection.
- A reduction in the number of platelets in the blood, which increases the risk of bleeding. Precautions must be taken to prevent injury.
- Destruction of the mucous membranes of the mouth. This causes burning, pain, redness, and breakdown inside the mouth.

Many other side effects are caused by chemotherapy drugs. The nurse will advise you what to watch for in each patient.

Disposal of Body Fluids and Wastes

Patients receiving chemotherapy may excrete the drugs in their waste and body fluids.

Discard gloves and other protective apparel, if worn, in a leakproof container. Follow facility policies for discarding in biohazardous waste or other area identified for contaminated materials. Because the drugs are excreted in body waste, linens that have contacted blood, body fluids, or excretions require special handling. Wear gloves when handling linen and always apply the principles of standard precautions. Soiled items should be bagged in specially marked bags before sending to the laundry.

Special Care of the Chemotherapy Patient

- Observe for and report side effects of the drugs to the nurse promptly.
- Provide nursing comfort measures, such as good mouth care, and daily bathing.
- Routinely take precautions to prevent injuries and infection.
- Take vital signs every 4 hours, or as ordered.
- Check with the nurse before taking a rectal temperature.
- Report a fever over 101°F or chilling to the nurse immediately. Other signs of infection to report are:
  - Swelling, redness, irritation inside the mouth
  - Rectal pain or tenderness
  - Change in bowel or bladder habits
  - Pain or burning on urination
  - Redness, swelling, open area, or pain on the skin
  - Cough or shortness of breath
  - Decreased level of consciousness
  - Decreased urine output
  - Warm, flushed, dry skin
  - Hypotension (below 100/60 mm Hg)

- Because of the risk of bleeding, patients may have to take special precautions, such as blowing the nose gently or using an electric razor.
- A very soft toothbrush will probably be necessary.
- Special mouthwash products may be ordered. The care plan and the nurse will provide specific directions.
- Promote good nutrition and hydration.
- The physician may order six small meals a day.
- High-protein drinks may also be ordered.
- Encourage fluids and record intake and output, including emesis.

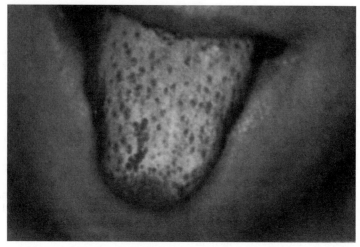

Figure 43-1 Monitor for and report white patches in the mouth to the nurse. (Courtesy of Daniel J. Barbaro, MD, Fort Worth, Texas)

- Alternate periods of rest with periods of activity to reduce fatigue.
- Plan your care to allow for frequent rest periods.

Inform the nurse if the patient:
- Has nausea or vomiting
- Is not eating or drinking
- Complains of changes in the taste buds affecting the ability or desire to eat
- Has constipation or diarrhea
- Has white patches or unusual areas inside the mouth (Figure 43-1)
- Complains of signs of a vaginal infection
- Develops bruising (Figure 43-2) or bleeding

Because chemotherapy drugs are so toxic, you must observe the patient closely when he or she is receiving them.

Inform the nurse promptly if the following appear:
- Signs of intravenous infiltration, such as redness, swelling, or pain at the needle insertion site

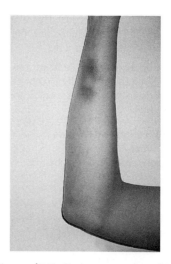

Figure 43-2 Bruises are a sign of internal bleeding. Report them promptly.

- Change in mental status
- Change in vital signs

Assisting the Patient with Body Image

Cancer surgery and chemotherapy may change body appearance, which often is very upsetting to the patient. Hair loss may be especially traumatic, particularly in females. Be calm and reassuring. The hair will grow back, although the color or texture may be different. Assist the patient to wear a turban, scarf, or wig, if desired.

Radiation Therapy

Radiation therapy involves the use of high-energy ionizing beams to the site of the cancer. The objective is to destroy the cancerous tissue without damaging healthy tissue. Several types of radiation therapy may be used.

Brachytherapy

Brachytherapy is a form of radiation therapy in which tiny radioactive seeds or pellets are implanted directly inside the body. It has fewer side effects than traditional radiation therapy and has proven successful for treating localized cancers. Treatment may last from several hours to several days. Depending on the location, the seeds may be left in place permanently. Brachytherapy may be used in combination with traditional radiation therapy.

Side Effects

Common side effects of radiation that should be reported to the nurse are:

- Fatigue
- Nausea, vomiting
- Diarrhea
- Skin redness, irritation, peeling
- Change in taste
- Irritation of mucous membranes
- Cough
- Shortness of breath

Special Care of the Radiation Therapy Patient

The patient may have markings on the skin at the site where radiation is delivered.

- Do not wash these off.
- The radiation may be very irritating to the patient's skin. Check the skin daily for problems and report them to the nurse, if found.
- Special skin care may be listed on the care plan, such as:
  - Washing the patient with luke-warm water and mild soap; in some situations no soap is used.
  - Avoiding rubbing or creating friction on the skin.
  - Avoiding shaving areas near the treatment field.
  - Avoiding tape on the patient's skin near the treatment field.
  - Avoiding lotions and cosmetics near the treatment field.
  - Avoiding tight-fitting garments; dress the patient in loose, comfortable clothing.

Protecting Yourself from Radiation Exposure

Sources of radiation are sometimes implanted inside the patient's body. If this is the case, you will be instructed in special precautions to follow to reduce your risk of radiation exposure (Figure 43-3). A list of precautions will be placed on the chart or elsewhere. Follow these instructions carefully. In general, you should:

- Inform the nurse if you are pregnant or suspect you may be pregnant.
- Not remain in the patient's room any longer than necessary.
- Stay at least 3 feet away from the patient unless direct care is being delivered.
- Find out if special precautions are necessary for handling soiled linens, tissues, or dressings.
- Wear the dosimeter to which you were assigned on the upper part of your body. The *dosimeter* is a small instrument that measures the radiation dose to which you are exposed

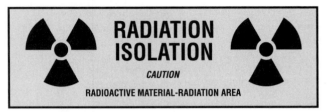

Figure 43-3 The radiation precautions sign has a black or magenta tri-blade on a white or yellow background, with the words "Caution: Radioactive Material." No one should enter the room without first consulting medical, nursing, or radiation safety staff.

when working with the patient. When you are off duty, store it according to facility policy. Do not take the badge home.

- If a radiation source becomes dislodged, avoid touching it. Ask visitors to leave the room. Try to move the source to a corner by using a tool, such as a yardstick. Inform the nurse or radiation safety personnel.

- Some brachytherapy seeds may be lost through urination. Strain the urine of patients who have seeds placed near the bladder. Follow facility policies for straining urine in a catheter bag. In some facilities, careful visual inspection of the catheter bag is sufficient. If a seed is found, do not attempt to remove it. Inform the nurse or radiation safety personnel.

- The instructions may vary slightly according to the type of treatment the patient is receiving. Become familiar with and follow the instructions on the care plan.

Immunotherapy

Immunotherapy is another cancer treatment that alters the patient's immune reaction and eliminate the cancer. Various biologic agents are given to change the normal immune response. The vital signs are regularly and closely monitored when these agents are given. Side effects of therapy usually cease within a week after treatment. Care of the patient receiving immunotherapy involves:

- Monitoring vital signs every 4 hours, or more often if instructed

- Monitoring capillary refill as instructed

- Advising the patient to remain in bed if the systolic blood pressure is below 100, or according to the nurse's instructions

- Weighing the patient daily and informing nurse of weight gain

Notify the nurse promptly if the patient:

- Has fever or chills

- Has rapid pulse (over 100, or according to nurse's instructions) or rapid respirations (over 24, or according to nurse's instructions)

- Becomes cyanotic

- Is short of breath

- Is restless, apprehensive

- Has diarrhea, nausea, or vomiting

- Complains of itching

PAIN

Pain is the most common symptom of patients with cancer. The pain may be caused by the cancer or as a result of the treatment. The pain may cause difficulty sleeping, loss of appetite, depression, and anxiety. Pain over an extended period of time reduces the patient's quality of life.

Cancer patients should be evaluated regularly for pain. A pain scale is usually used. Narcotic pain-relieving medications may be necessary to control the pain. These are not withheld out of fear of addiction. The incidence of addiction is very low. Pain should be treated before it becomes severe and out of control. Notify the nurse promptly if a patient complains of pain.

MENTAL AND EMOTIONAL NEEDS

Patients with cancer have a life-altering disease. They often fear dying and may be anxious or depressed. They often go through the grieving process. Nursing assistant measures to assist with mental and emotional needs include:

- Spending as much time as possible with the patient if he or she wants to talk
- Allowing the patient to talk about feelings and fears
- Being proficient at providing physical care and assistance with ADLs
- Anticipating patients' needs before they ask
- Respecting the patient's beliefs and wishes

- Providing emotional support
- Respecting the patient's privacy if he or she wants to be alone
- Making the patient feel respected and valued as a person

Avoid giving the patient false hope. If you think a patient is losing control, inform the nurse. Just being with the patient and allowing him or her to talk is very helpful.

PALLIATIVE CARE

Some patients with cancer elect to have palliative care, which is designed to treat the symptoms of discomfort but not the disease. The patient will have an advance directive and a do not resuscitate order. He or she is kept comfortable until death occurs. A hospice may be involved in the patient's care. One goal of this care is to maintain the patient's quality of life for as long as possible.

Nursing Assistant Measures

Your care is designed to keep the patient clean and comfortable. Use nursing measures, such as positioning and backrubs, to enhance the patient's comfort. Spend time with the patient and allow him or her to talk, if desired. Respect the patient's wishes. Provide emotional support. Inform the nurse if the patient is short of breath, is anxious, or complains of pain.

INDEX